THE HE

A Star Original

Peter Lambley has lectured on Psychology, and psychological medicine at the University of Cape Town. He has published several papers on migraine and on various aspects of psychology as well as many magazine articles.

THE HEADACHE BOOK
A Self-Help Guide for Headache and Migraine Sufferers

Dr Peter Lambley

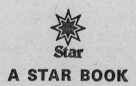

A STAR BOOK

published by
the Paperback Division of
W. H. ALLEN & Co. Ltd

A Star Book
Published in 1980
by the Paperback Division of
W. H. Allen & Co. Ltd
A Howard and Wyndham Company
44 Hill Street, London W1X 8LB

Copyright © Peter Lambley 1980

Printed in Great Britain by
Hunt Barnard Printing Ltd., Aylesbury, Bucks.

ISBN 0352 30647 5

Contents

Chapter 1	Introduction	7
Chapter 2	Finding your way	9
Chapter 3	Who gets headaches?	18
Chapter 4	What is headache?	28
Chapter 5	When are headaches dangerous?	41
Chapter 6	What causes headache?	51
Chapter 7	Headache as a psychosomatic problem	61
Chapter 8	Migraine people	73
Chapter 9	Treatment 1: Muscle-contraction (tension) headache	88
Chapter 10	Treatment 2: Migraine	104
Chapter 11	Towards a cure 1: Concepts, diagnosis and the mild headache	118
Chapter 12	Towards a cure 2: Moderate-interference headache	141
Chapter 13	Towards a cure 3: Major or chronic-interference headache	158
Glossary		165
References		168

Acknowledgements

I would like to thank Dorrian McLaren, Amalia Tziairis, Shelley Power, Derek Mullis of the Migraine Trust and my patients for the help they provided in preparing this book. I also gratefully acknowledge the assistance of the staff of the University of Athens Medical School library. The opinions expressed, however, are solely my own except where otherwise stated.

CHAPTER ONE

Introduction

This is a book about headaches. It takes them, examines them and tells you what they are, what they mean, why they happen and what to do about them. It tells you about ordinary headache, about migraine and all its variants, and it tells you about dangerous headaches and how to tell them from safe ones. When all that is done it takes the field apart – examining how headaches are treated by drugs, by behaviour therapy, psychotherapy, surgery, even acupuncture. It looks at theories and ideas about headache and it tries to weigh them up, to proportion out heredity and environment, psychology and neurology, to give a proper perspective of things as they stand now.

Nothing in this book is incomprehensible, nothing is too technical or too medical. Deliberately so. You, the ordinary person, need to know where you stand and where the professionals stand. I am a professional and I have worked with, treated and done research on headache sufferers. I also get occasional headaches myself and, as an adolescent, had migraine. What I have tried to do in this book is to give *you* the kind of information *I* would have wanted to know myself when I first began to get headache and if now, as a professional, I wanted to know accurately about the state of someone else's speciality. I would hate to be duped, treated like a fool or fobbed off with treatments that were less than useless, and I have presumed you feel the same.

By the same token, I haven't spared anyone's feelings when it comes to the personality of the headache sufferer or where I think they contribute needlessly to their own problems. In trying to be fair and objective, there is no point in being polite to one another, whoever you may be.

A large proportion of this book is devoted to spelling out what *you*, the sufferer, can realistically do about your headache. There are literally hundreds of ways in which you can contribute to making things better for yourself and these are detailed where appropriate. The last three chapters, however, tell you how to organise your own treatment and to work towards a cure with or without help. Again, the emphasis is on all of us, sufferer and doctor alike, working and researching towards a cure. Keep an open mind, think carefully, don't expect an easy answer, and we could all be in business. Good hunting.

CHAPTER TWO

Finding your way

Headaches are no fun. They hit you when the *last* thing you need after a simply terrible day is a nagging, throbbing pain in the head that refuses to go away. Or you can be busy, in a rush with a million important things to do and it's still only lunch time when you realise that the tight feeling across your brow has been with you for the past hour and is not getting any better. Worse, headaches are infuriatingly indiscriminate. Just when you're set to go out and relax, to enjoy yourself after a hard week at work or at home with the kids, when there is really no reason why you should be physically strung up, along comes that strange removed feeling which means you're in for a migraine attack. There is no surer way of ruining a promising weekend, not only for the sufferer, but for the rest of the family as well.

You can take some comfort. Headaches have been around a long time. As early as 3,000 BC, the term 'sick-headed' was in use while stone tablets at Epidaurus dating from 400 BC describe a case of insomnia due to headaches. Both Socrates and Plato in the fourth century BC were aware of the relationship between being tense or upset and headache; while Soranus of Ephesus, a Greek physician practising in Rome in the second century AD, wrote surprisingly informative descriptions of both chronic headache and migraine.

So, for something like 5,000 years, men and women have been plagued by headaches. In fact, after hunger and fatigue, they have been for centuries the most common and the most distressing physical complaint, interfering with the conquests and careers of both Julius Caesar and Alexander the Great as well as the thoughts of Rudyard Kipling and Lewis Carroll. And, of course, people – famous or otherwise – still suffer from headaches today.

Unlike other areas of medical research, the treatment of headache and migraine has not greatly benefited from the enormous advances made in science and technology. While we now know a great deal more about different kinds of headache and can reduce the pain of attacks considerably, we are no nearer a cure for them than Hippocrates or Soranus were. To be frank, we still do not know properly what *causes* headache and migraine, which is, of course, the kind of admission that embarrasses all medical scientists. Admitting that the causes of cancer are as yet unknown is one thing. To say the same about even the most simple and straightforward of headaches – such commonplace and medically insignificant events – is to eat humble pie indeed.

The difficulty is that headache like the mysterious common cold isn't serious enough as a medical or human problem to warrant or attract the kind of massive attention that cancer or heart disease has. Worse, headache, unlike the common cold, has widely been presumed to be a psychological phenomenon. Unfortunately, for centuries, anything said to be 'emotional' or to take place 'in the mind' was not taken seriously. It has only been because migraine – the hard edge, as it were, of the headache syndrome – can be such a debilitating experience that researchers in the last two centuries have turned their interest to headache, helped, no doubt, by wealthy or prominent patrons afflicted by it. Even today, most medical and scientific reports on headache focus on migraine, despite the fact that migraine accounts for only 20 per cent of all reported headaches.

Of course, the kiss of death from physical medicine usually means the kiss of life for psychology or psychiatry. One man's meat is another man's poison. No sooner is a disorder excluded from the realm of physical medicine than every psychoanalyst, psychiatrist and psychologist within miles picks it up and 'saves' it by breathing symbolic meaning into it. Usually the 'disorder' succumbs eventually under the many years of 'penetrating' analysis. Fortunately for headache, it has not suffered as a disorder from the worse effects of these psychologising processes. It was picked up – especially when psychoanalysis and its related disciplines were at their height in the 1940s and 1950s – but it was very quickly dropped like a hot brick when it was discovered that no amount of symbolising or analysis actually stopped the patient from getting headache. To *cure* does not mean to give symbolism, sympathy or a pain killer. It is to remove the occurrence of the illness and, in this, headache has eluded the best efforts of physicians, surgeons and psychiatrists alike for something like fifty centuries. A sobering thought indeed.

You can see, then, that headache has been something rather more than just an embarrassment. So you may wonder what, if anything, is the point of reading a book about headaches if nobody can cure them. This is just the point at which this book begins. It would be foolish and dishonest to start off by promising help or cures that simply don't exist or by painting a rosy picture of our current knowledge that is little more than a figment of our collective medical imaginations. Headache is a problem and I believe we must, all of us, doctors and laymen alike start from a realistic appreciation of what we, the doctors, *do* know, and what we *can* do, and what you, the sufferers, *experience*. The aim of this book is to go on from a realistic assessment of headache to have a look at what *you*, the sufferer, can realistically do to help yourself and help your doctor or physician work for you better.

Now before you dismiss this with a shrug and think 'Oh, another of those "be good little patients" advice books' or if your attitude is of the 'well if doctors can't fix them how the bloody hell can we?' type, wait a minute. If you suffer from headache, then you may be surprised to learn that it is the one illness in which the patient has a *better* chance, at the moment and for the forseeable future, than either his or her general practitioner or medical researchers of finding a cure for their own particular syndrome. Assuming that your head-ache is not caused by an organic or infectious illness – and most of them are not – then, *nobody* knows your headache and what causes it *better* than you do. What you need most and what this book is about is help, advice and guidance on how to go about finding out about your particular problem. Knowing where to look and what to look for can help you manage your own psychology and physical health better. Let me explain.

There are basically three types of headache. The first and by far the most frequently occurring is headache caused by social and psychological stress – you get tense, tired, upset, irritable and the result is a headache. The second, less psychological in origin, is caused by a variety of physical stresses and some medical problems. You can get headache from eyestrain, from certain kinds of dental problems and sinusitus, from eat-ing certain kinds of food, from certain minor infections, from certain drugs, from lack of sleep, from swimming in ice-cold water, and so on. These are all essentially physical things which contribute to or precipitate headache.

Lastly, you can get headache from more serious organic or physical events. You get a painful headache if you're hit on the head by a brick, if you have a brain haemorrhage or tumour, and from serious infections like meningitis or encephalitis (an inflammation of the brain). Fortunately, this last category forms a relatively low percentage of reported headaches and often has fairly obvious accompanying symptoms or causes.

Of the three, the first occurs most commonly and this is where you and your mental processes come in. *Who* you are, how you behave, what you think and feel and, above all, how you react to *stress* are the central factors that help to cause these kinds of headache, and this includes tension or muscle-contraction headache, migraine and 'cluster' headache. We may not know yet quite why the individual creates his or her own headache but we do know that a large part of the cause may well lie in the individual's emotional life and therefore, logically, treatment and cure should be found in the same area.

There are those who would argue against this view. They would say that headaches are essentially a physical reaction involving higher brain functions (or, rather, dysfunctions) that have nothing to do with psychology. There are other people who argue that headaches, especially migraine, are inherited – if your parents got them, so will you and there is little you can do about them. After all, you can't fight the cells or muscles and bones that make up your body, can you? Or can you?

Well, yes, you can. In certain respects, anyway. The one thing that modern medical and physiological research has clearly substantiated is the almost incredible flexibility of the human physical system – especially the functions of the brain and its surrounding grey matter, the cerebral cortex. It used to be thought that each part of the brain had a specific function and that you inherited a capacity or organisation of each of these functions. If you lost a function – through injury, perhaps, or if you suffered a certain indisposition, like headache – it was because you had an 'inherited weakness' of these specific areas.

Well, as you may have noticed, there have been rather a lot of wars this century in which rather a lot of people suffered injury to the head or to the brain. Thanks to this and to the advent of the scientific era, we know now that while the brain does have specific areas that serve specific functions, many of these areas can receive quite extensive damage or destruction without the brain as a whole ceasing to perform the function usually associated with that area. Like a good rugby team that loses a couple of men – so long as they aren't Gareth Edwards and Phil Bennet – the brain somehow copes by sharing the work burden around among undamaged areas. If the damaged brain can do this, think of what the undamaged, relatively healthy brain can do.

Quite apart from the fact that these discoveries revolutionised both our thinking about and knowledge of brain functioning, they helped to put the position and importance of genetically inherited disorders and physical abilities in a better perspective. You may well inherit a tendency or capacity but what you do *after* you have inherited it is very much a function of *you* and your interaction with your environment. If you inherit, for example, a curable blood disease and you and your doctor know about it, you can often, either by having a timely transfusion or taking appropriate measures, prevent yourself from *ever* having an attack of the disease. Since some diseases become incurable after a certain time has elapsed, the act of spotting and recognising the symptoms in time can save your life. I need hardly add that the act of recognition is certainly not an inherited or physically determined one, it often depends on you or the skill of your doctor.

By the same token – and taking the argument a little further – you can inherit the best intelligence in the world (intelligence is also supposed to be genetically determined) but if you also happen to be paranoid or withdrawn or depressed or suffer from an inferiority complex, you may never get to use your intelligence. How often have we read on a child's school report: 'Has intelligence but emotional and personal factors interfere with it.'?

And so it is for the headache. Whether or not headache will be found to have a simple biochemical cause or to be inherited does not affect the role played by the individual in their control and maintenance. If the brain can override specific disorders to continue functioning well, so then can the individual direct his or her mental functioning to ensure that this natural brain flexibility and resilience is carried through to the level of social and personal day-to-day living. Simply put, even if headaches are inherited, you may be able to overcome them.

In fact, many people who suffer from recurring headaches try to do just that. Ask any chronic sufferer of headaches how they help themselves and you will get an insight into a world of functioning and a level of experience you didn't know existed. Many sufferers have well-established private rituals, not prescribed by their physicians, either to avoid getting a headache or to minimise the pain. One patient of mine avoided looking at brightly coloured objects because he sensed they

14

precipitated his migraine. Whether he was justified medically or not, if he did by chance look at a bright colour, migraine inevitably followed and, if he didn't – it didn't. Another patient never raised his eyes upward. Heaven knows how he avoided accidents from falling objects but, he claimed, it did prevent headaches. In the headache literature there is a report of one migraine sufferer who aborted his attacks by eating copious quantities of pasta. Presumably he preferred being overweight to having migraine. In another case of mine, a football-playing fanatic had cured his migraine, which seemed to come on in the middle of a game, by playing in very dark glasses. Alas, he was a goalkeeper and his career suffered. Again though his inventiveness did, he claims, reduce his headache attacks.

The point is that self-help of this kind has its limitations. Chronic headache sufferers use a great deal of ingenuity in helping themselves but it is seldom in the right area. My goal-keeping patient's system may have been efficient in reducing his attacks but, believe me – and I have this direct from his captain – it ruined his game. Many migraine patients become so involved in trying to minimise or prevent their attacks that they have little time or energy left over to enjoy their lives or to form adequate and fulfilling relationships, neglecting their spouses, their children and, ultimately, themselves.

One of the reasons for this general inefficiency lies in the way people think and are informed about headache. There is a general tendency, for example, for doctors – especially busy G.P.s – to dismiss headache as a mere 'mental' problem. They tell patients to relax and take life easy and, at best, prescribe a tranquilliser, quite unaware of the inadequacy both of this advice and of the biochemical action of the medicine given. The patient goes away, tries unsuccessfully to relax, takes the unhelpful pill and eventually gives up and puts up with his or her headache, carrying on an elaborate avoidance system.

The general ethic of our drug-orientated culture doesn't help either. The public is routinely exposed to the idea that medicine has advanced amazingly to cure every and all possible problems. No wonder the disillusioned headache patient prefers to sit it out and wait. After all, hundreds of new pills appear on the market every month and any one of them may provide the promised cure.

It is this attitude of easy dismissal of headache as either a minor or irrelevant or psychological problem combined with the promise of a drug-based utopia around the corner that does the most harm to the ordinary person's comprehension of headache phenomena. Sadly, if he or she decides to seek alternative advice, say from a psychologist or psychiatrist, life can sometimes be made a lot worse. Many psychologists and psychiatrists explore areas of personal functioning and pathology that are only dimly relevant to the problem of headache. In the end they can be as inefficiently irrelevant as the G.P.'s tranquilliser and his advice to relax. This is one of the reasons that some G.P.s are not keen to refer patients to psychiatrists. It is better, they argue, to live with the pain you know than with that which you didn't know existed.

The right answer, as always, lies somewhere buried amidst this plethora of good intentions and sound advice. The doctor who tells his patient to relax is pointing in the right direction, as too is the assistance that he and psychiatrists and psychologists give. The headache sufferer who tries to help her or himself by taking little physical and psychological precautions is also taking steps in the right direction, but none of them are either efficient or enough. What I want to do in this book is to help point you, the sufferer, in the right direction, to improve your efficiency and, hopefully, to launch you on to the path of cure. Believe me, if anyone is going to find it for you, you are.

First, we will see who suffers from headache and how widespread they are. Then we will discuss the three kinds of headache so that you know what kind of headache *you* get, what symptoms are associated with each and, briefly, how they arise. Then we'll have a look at serious or dangerous headache just so you'll know if it happens to you or to someone in your family. We'll also have a look at headache and migraine in children and adolescents to help parents spot earlier if their children have problems.

After that, we'll look at the mechanisms of headache, how they are caused. The experience of headache is principally a matter of physiology. The blood vessels in your head contract and this causes the pain, but how and why they contract is both interesting and fascinating. Physiological changes are linked to one another and to your personality in an intriguing way to set up the social, psychological and physical circumstances that cause headache. In Chapter 7 we will start untangling this complex interaction and look at the steps that can be taken to minimise or prevent headache.

Before we go to specific therapies, we have a look in Chapter 8 at migraine, the Big Brother of all headaches. Finally, in the last three chapters, we'll examine treatments, medical, physiological and psychological. At each stage, we will relate them both to the mechanisms involved (discussed in Chapters 6 and 7) and to the self-help programme we develop throughout the book.

Reading the book isn't going to turn you into a headache expert. But it is going to make you a lot wiser about your own pattern and it is, I feel sure, going to stimulate you into experimenting with your own psychology. Even if you don't want to change parts of your personality or your social behaviour, the book will help you to use medication better, to help you ride *with* a painkiller, for example, and not against it, and to guard against over-doses or using the wrong kind of medication for your personality or circumstances.

I believe that one wise and well-informed patient is worth a score of uninformed patients. It is a tremendous help to a doctor and a patient who can actively participate in his or her own treatment saves an awful lot of time and trouble. Being wise about headaches is, after 5,000 years of trying, something that human beings could well afford to value.

CHAPTER THREE

Who gets headaches?

The popular image of the headache sufferer, especially of the migraine sufferer, is of a highly intelligent, even brilliant person whose high level of intellect and creativity is paid for in the frequency of the accompanying headache. We are all familiar with the notion of the artist or Great Man or Woman struggling with a Great Idea having periodic headaches as the strain gets too much. Like a woman undergoing labour pains in order to give birth to a child, we easily see the connection between the two and treat it with respect. The list of famous and great people who suffered from migraine or headache is sufficiently long and impressive to firmly cement this view in our minds. After all, if Napoleon and George Bernard Shaw suffered from headaches, what more proof do you need?

The difficulty with this notion is that the opposite is not true: that is, if geniuses and highly intelligent people get headache, it should follow that the ordinary person, the average Jill or Johnny, does not get headache or migraine. He or she is – or should be – blithely ignorant of 'higher things' and, as a reward, travel through life quite undisturbed by head pain. What most headache researchers are generally agreed upon (and there is precious little agreement amongst them) is that just about *everyone* gets simple headache at one time or another during their lifetime and that literally millions of people suffer from more severe headache of a recurring kind.

In the United States, for example, it was estimated in the late 1960s that between 12 and 25 million Americans suffer from severe headache, a figure that is in reality now probably much higher due to population increase and to the fact that we are now much more aware of how research studies and estimates tap only the tip of the iceberg.

In Britain, it is estimated that something like 15 to 20 per cent of adult men and 24 to 29 per cent of adult women suffer from migraine (Waters, 1975). Since migraine is the more severe form of headache it is quite likely that the percentage of people who suffer from general headaches is much higher*: something like 30 million adult Britons of both sexes. They can't all be geniuses, can they?

More sobering still for those who would like to believe that only the intelligent get headache are the results of a very thorough scientific study done by W. E. Waters in 1968. Studying adults in the Pontypridd parliamentary constituency in Wales, he compared the intelligence of migraine sufferers with that of non-migraine sufferers and with people who got headache but not migraine. He found no evidence that migraine, or indeed headache sufferers as a whole, were more intelligent than their headache-free fellow constituents. What he did find, though, was that the more intelligent migraine sufferer was more likely to see a doctor about his or her migraine than the less intelligent migraine sufferer, indicating that doctors and clinics that *treat* headache may well have gained the impression that migraine patients were on the average more intelligent. So there you have it.

The real question about who gets headache should, I think, really be 'who *doesn't* get headache?' One study I conducted among a small student sample (small in number, not stature) failed to find a *single* person, male or female, who had not had headache. Most (over 80 per cent) had at least one fairly severe headache a month which accords fairly well with the available research literature. In a major study conducted in the early fifties in New Orleans, Louisiana, one of the highest incidences of headache was recorded in university first-year students and

* Green (1975) found 28 per cent of Members of Parliament to suffer from migraine and in a large sample of Britons (just under 15,000), nearly 20 per cent of males and 25 per cent of females.

in medical students, 86 per cent of whom suffered from headache. Nearly 50 per cent of the 4,634 people who took part in the study had more than one headache a month and 65 per cent had periodic headaches.

What does seem to be true though, is that people who live in rural areas get less headaches than those who live in cities and older people seem to suffer less than young. The New Orleans study found the lowest incidence of headache amongst male Negro labourers of whom only 8 per cent of those studied got them (white labourers had twice the incidence). But before you latch on to the racial theme, Negro nuns had, in the same study, the highest incidence (87 per cent) of headache. So, look elsewhere for an explanation.

Social class, incidentally, is another headache myth that must be dispensed with and one that will, hopefully, disappear in time from our folklore. *Top* people do not get migraine any more than *bottom* people do. The Pontypridd Survey found no indication that people of social class I and II (the top two of the five classes used in research by social scientists) had a higher incidence of migraine than the other classes. Again though, it was found that 'top' people were more likely to consult a doctor about their headache than 'bottom' people – hence the impression gained by such notable medical authorities as Dr Fothergill in the eighteenth century and Dr Day in the nineteenth. The latter, for example, wrote an influential text book on headache in which he described the headache sufferer as being highly cultured, of nervous and delicate disposition and possessor of a vivid imagination, which may be nice but not, unfortunately, true. In much the same way the highly civilised and highly cultured Athenians of Ancient Greece, who took headache cures at sanctuaries founded by Hippocrates under the aegis of the god Aescupios, were *efpatrides* (privileged citizens). Poorer people couldn't afford the luxury too often, and slaves . . . well, you know how they treated slaves.

The most solidly consistent finding that has withstood the tests of both time and the twentieth century is that women more than men get headaches. It is estimated that between twice as many and four times as many women suffer from headache than men. Quite why this is so is not so well established. Much has been made of the role of menstruation and some experts have attributed the tendency of many women to develop headache or migraine before or around their menstrual period to the drop in levels of certain hormones, primarily oestrogen (Somerville, 1972). Since these changes are more frequent and regular in women, it has been argued that this may account for the higher incidence of headache in women.

There are other considerations, though. Not all women get headache or migraine with their periods or during ovulation, a fact that greatly reduces the sweeping statements about the menstruation link. If lowered levels of hormones is the cause of excessive headache in females, it should theoretically be true of nearly all women. And not all women get headache. Much more research needs to be done on this before we will be able to clarify the hormonal picture further.

One hypothesis that deserves consideration to explain the higher incidence in females – and take the self-satisfied smile off male readers' faces – is that given the social role and status of women in modern societies, it is very likely that women will more often feel social approval for the expression of pain or discomfort than men will. Men tend to suffer from the S.U.L.C. syndrome* and keep their pain to themselves, in the process inflicting painful emotional internal damage to themselves and to others. Women, it seems, are much more likely to inflict their doctors and anyone who will listen with their expressions of distress. Since women generally live longer than men and have a higher tolerance of pain, the statistics on female headache may well be telling us something very fundamental both about headache and how to deal with them – but more about that in a later chapter.

* Stiff Upper Lip and Cranium syndrome, also known amongst headache habitués as the 'Grin and Bear it' outlook and the 'Turn your face to the wall' mentality.

Suffice it to say for now that women may get headaches more often than men because they tend to use headache as a means of expressing their anger and frustration about their lot in life. Women are allowed to be more *emotional* than men, but they aren't permitted to do as much *about* their distress as men can. A man can always – and many do – bury his frustrations by driving like a maniac, drinking more than he should, fooling around with his friends and in general, get away from it all much easier than women. Women are far more tied by their social roles, their families and their sense of inadequacy than men are. There is some evidence to suggest that men who get headache are more sensitive, less 'macho' and less male-stereotyped than males who don't get headache. The inference is that these men either are not satisfied by the normal male expressions of frustration or that they fear condemnation for being like the 'macho' males currently under attack by the feminist media. This hypothesis may not be so far-fetched as it sounds. There is some indication that male headache sufferers are generally closer to their mothers, or are reared in homes in which the female figures are more dominant, than non-headache males. The same psychological mechanism that may account for the higher incidence in females may also well account, in part, for the reason many men get headache.

Women apart, headaches are consistently reported in certain occupation groups more than others. People who work in conditions which expose them to high levels of carbon monoxide gas, for example (one of the dangerous elements in car exhaust fumes that are in the process of being phased out by car manufacturers), are liable to get painful vascular headaches caused by irritation in the blood vessels. People who work with or near poisons like lead, carbon tetrachloride, benzene, insecticides and so on, are affected in the same way.

There are other risky occupations. I once visited the home of a friend whose uncle was staying with them. After a while I was struck by the obsessional and obviously neurotic relationship my friend's uncle had with his hat. He never took it off, inside or outside the house, at mealtimes, even going to the toilet. Eventually I couldn't resist it any longer.

'Do you sleep in your hat?' I asked as noncommitally as I could using a manner I generally adopt with chronic psychotic patients when inquiring about their delusions.

'Oh no,' he said, quite unperturbed. 'I take it off and wear a head band.'

This man, I subsequently discovered, worked in a dynamite factory and was on holiday. He wore a hat and the head band because on both, around the inner lining, he had rubbed some traces of dynamite mixture. If he didn't do this, when he returned to work after a break, his renewed daily contact with the nitrates used in dynamite production would give him the most excruciating headache that could last a week. Since workers quickly adapt to the stuff, it is obviously better for them to keep some around even when on holiday to avoid these headaches. Don't worry, the quantity smeared on their hats is minute and not dangerous. And of course, you can't explode dynamite without a detonator. If you see a dynamite worker with a detonator stuck in his hatband, however, proceed with caution.

People who are exposed to strains in their jobs, like air traffic controllers, appear to develop unpleasant things such as hypertension. Whether or not people in these occupations also develop headache is unclear. Of course, there are many environmental events that are presumed to cause migraine – noise, intense or flickering light, poor ventilation, heat, eyestrain, the weather – but these may simply *precipitate* attacks rather than actually *cause* migraine. Some people work and live quite happily under the most trying of environmental stresses without getting even the faintest glimmer of a headache. Other people get migraine when they are *away* from the job – over the weekend or on holiday. The Pontypridd survey found, for example, that most migraines are recorded on Saturday and Sunday and the fewest on Monday. Since the researchers also found that migraines most commonly occur between lunchtime and eight o'clock at night, one is tempted in fact to say that it does rather look as if going to work on

Monday morning cures migraine while thoughts of going home each day (presumably occurring from lunchtime onwards) or actually being at home (over the weekend) are almost certain guarantees of getting a migraine attack. Food for thought, indeed.

Talking of food, some people who love eating certain types of food can also get headaches. Believe it or not, eating ice-cream can give some people quite a nasty headache, so too can over-indulgence in Chinese foods (the Chinese Restaurant Syndrome, as it's known to the cogniscenti). Hot dogs, bacon, salami and ham, chocolates, oranges, tomatoes, onions, pine-apples and fatty foods, eating ripe cheeses while on certain psychiatric drugs, can all cause headache. Missing a meal can give you a headache. Of course, people who drink too much alcohol may get a hangover headache. Too much coffee, as well as suddenly stopping the habit of drinking coffee, may give you a headache. And marijuana smokers sometimes also report mild headaches in the front regions of their heads. I know of no data on headache with chronic heroin users but possibly they wouldn't notice one way or another.

Children get headache, usually in conjunction with one or another of the childhood fevers and illnesses. Tonsillitis, influenza, measles and mumps cause particularly intense head-aches as can the more serious illnesses like polio, pneumonia and septicemia. Children can also get headaches in connection with general anxiety about school, homework, teachers and so on. Epileptic fits in children sometimes produce headache along with other symptoms, particularly gastro-intestinal dis-turbances and have to be carefully differentiated from migraine attacks. We'll deal with this – and indeed with all the other types – later in the book. Surprisingly enough, children are now thought to get migraine or migraine-like disturbances about which, more later.

For a long time, it was thought (and still is in many quar-ters) that headache – especially migraine – ran in families. If your father or mother had migraine, for example, then there was a good chance that you too would suffer from it. The probability, according to some researchers, is as high as 90 per cent (Bakal, 1975). If you are a twin and your family has a history of migraine, then, according to Refsum (1968), there's a 60 to 100 per cent chance that your twin and you will have migraine – assuming you are mono-zygotic twins (that is, from the same egg). The percentages drop to between 10 and 40 per cent for dizygotic (different egg) twins. The trouble is that this theory of genetic inheritance does not stand up too well under conditions of proper scientific assessment. To go back to the Pontypridd study again, the prevalence of migraine was only 5 and 6 per cent in the families of the headache and headache-free groups studied, respectively, and only 10 per cent in the families of migraine sufferers. As the author of the survey points out, this suggests that far too much emphasis has been placed on the hereditary nature of migraine. His figures back him up almost to the hilt; while it is more likely that you will have migraine if your family has a history of it than if it doesn't, that likelihood is quite small.

My experience with migraine families leads me to suspect that having a parent or relative with a migraine or headache problem often helps the family in general to 'explain' their children's headaches, without probing too deeply into the real reasons why the child develops them. This is especially the case, I think, in migraine, where the condition in children is often preceded by a kind of confused agitation that is not found so clearly in adults. As we will see later, migraine may be a physical reaction to emotional confusion, the extent of which neither the person nor his family appreciates. The same reaction so clearly seen in childhood migraine may well disappear or, rather, become unattended to, as the child grows older because his or her attacks are 'explained' as being 'like aunty Mary's headaches'. I have found in clinical practice that migraine sufferers who came from families with no history of migraine tend to be far more ready to accept the idea that emotional factors may contribute to their headache frequency than those with well-established family histories. They will often in fact quite spontaneously pop up with something like:

'That's exactly what my mother said – she said I got headaches because I was upset about my exams but of course, nobody listened to her.' Having headaches, in some families with long histories of them, is as natural as brushing your teeth – you accept them and put up with them without question, a sad but true comment on the power of ignorance.

What probably helps to maintain this kind of quiet acceptance and almost masochistic ability to put up routinely with quite debilitating pain is the well-known and quite well-established personality qualities of headache sufferers. If you are tense, driving, obsessional, perfectionist, inflexible, defensive in an anxious way, achievement-orientated, hypersensitive to personal – or indeed any form of – criticism, intolerant, conventional, over-controlled and over-routined, there is a very strong chance that you suffer from headache or migraine. The more of these qualities you possess, the more likely your headaches are to take a severe form. I have heard it whispered privately by some medical practitioners that they have a check list of all these items and if a new patient exhibits all of the items in the first five minutes of the first consultation, the doctor just *knows* they have a migraine.

Seriously though, these kinds of qualities aren't usually associated with either personal insight or an ability to tolerate weakness in self or others, and these factors may well account for or at least contribute towards the maintenance and perhaps even the development of headaches. Since personal qualities such as these are usually learnt in the family, it follows that families with histories of headache or migraine may well be over-achievers, highly controlled and the like.

If this is the case and there is some indication that it is, then it suggests that children may get headaches as the only tolerated means of registering 'weakness'. A headache, because it is physical and therefore 'respectable', is permissible – crying or being upset at the pressures placed on you is not. More food for thought. For further developments, see chapters nine and ten.

What, finally, you may ask, do headaches cost us? The

26

answer is quite staggering. In 1962, the United States Public Health Service estimated that Americans spent about 300 million dollars annually on popular headache remedies, a figure, you will appreciate, that is now very much higher. In Britain, migraine cost the National Health Service alone £2.8 million in 1970, £1.6 million of that being spent on pharmaceuticals, the rest on general practice and hospital in-patient services (Pearce, 1975). The figures for private spending – ie, for tablets and aspirin bought without prescription or with a private doctor's prescription – are not available. If, however, we extrapolate from the old, out-of-date American figures for 1962, in which every American man, woman and child spent at least a dollar a year on headaches and even if we halve that rate to give the British population a conservative, less drug-prone bent which they may or may not possess, this still works out at something like £15 million spent annually on headache. An expensive business. Add to this the cost of work hours lost through headache (295,000 man hours and 167,000 woman hours in Britain in 1968–9 – a very conservative estimate), inefficiency, accidents, carelessness and emotional distress and the like, and you get an idea of just how big a phenomenon headache has become. It is a problem that certainly mustn't be underestimated.

One last word: medical and psychiatric patients are among the population groups who, understandably, experience more headaches than most people. Yet strangely enough, psychotic patients, the most severely disturbed of mental patients, such as schizophrenics, don't as a rule suffer excessively from headache. They sometimes complain of imaginary head pains and headaches which are part of their mental illness but, by and large, they are relatively headache-free.

Strange, isn't it, that while the rest of us rush around suffering from migraine and headache and all the other stresses and cares of living in the real world, the truly insane live undisturbed by headache. There's a moral in this somewhere . . .

CHAPTER FOUR

What is headache?

Having settled the preliminaries, we can now turn to examine headaches themselves and see just exactly what they are. Earlier, you will remember, we distinguished three broad types: headaches of essentially social or psychological origin, headaches of a physical or benign organic origin (that is, not organically serious in themselves) and headaches of a more severe organic or medical origin. In this chapter, we will focus on the first two types and go on to discuss the third type, potentially dangerous headache, in the next chapter.

First, though, let us be clear about what we are doing here. We will concern ourselves, in the next two chapters, with descriptive explanations of headache in contrast to the causes of headache, which we will examine from chapter five onwards. This may seem like a trivial point but it is a vital one for the reader to understand. Much of the confusion that has arisen about headache, not only in the minds of the public but in the minds of some doctors and scientists doing research, occurs because people confuse a causal explanation with a descriptive explanation. If I have a bad bruise on my arm and someone asks, 'What on earth is that black and blue thing?', a *descriptive* explanation would be something like: 'Oh, it's a bruise. The swelling and the colour is caused by damaged blood vessels and tissues under the skin'; while a *causal* explanation would be: 'I hit my arm with a hammer.' Both are really necessary for a full explanation, to explain every step between what you see and what happened, but it would obviously be foolish to 'explain' the bruise by saying it was 'caused' by the skin tissues. Unfortunately, however, this is just what happens sometimes in headache: people explain them by referring to descriptive explanations *as if they were causal ones*.

Let's examine briefly how this arises in headache. In order to get a *head* ache, certain things have to happen to the blood supply and its circulation to the brain. The brain itself is not sensitive to pain. Pain is experienced by the person mainly through the blood vessels, particularly through the arteries that feed blood to the brain and the large veins and venous sinuses that drain it out again. Blood is carried from the heart to the rest of the body that needs it – to muscles and the vital organs – by arteries. Anything that has an effect on this brain blood supply can cause pain to be registered on the pain receptors in the arteries and veins involved. This is a perfectly ordinary descriptive explanation but too many people stop there and treat headaches as if there is nothing else to them. This attitude is helped along by the fact that most pain killers seem to operate where the pain occurs, thus seeming to prove a cause-and-effect idea. It is a simple step from accepting this to accepting facile medical or paramedical 'causal' explanations that miss out a whole range of intermediary steps, not only in the brain but in the functioning of the individual both as a biological and a psychological being. Seeing headache as being a hereditary complaint or 'explaining' headache as a 'constitutional' weakness, or to say someone has – literally – 'sensitive' arteries, are short cuts all too often employed by both doctors and laymen who are not willing to go into the problems properly. This is as bad, in my opinion, as Freud's earlier suggestion that headaches of a psychological origin arise as a form of reaction to ideas of symbolic rape or, as he put it, defloration (Fine, 1969).

The real state of affairs, as you may have guessed, is that we know the real *cause* of headache in only a few very specific and mainly organic instances. We don't know what causes the major and most frequently experienced types of headache – migraine and tension headache. This is why it is so much easier to use simple explanations that sound either authentic or

29

medically sophisticated enough to put off all but the most determined of inquiries.

So, to avoid this pitfall, let us be clear that we are mainly concerning ourselves in this chapter with *descriptions* of headache and not causal explanations. Where a certain specific headache has a well-established cause, this will be clearly stated.

Head pain, as we have said, is most often a phenomenon associated with pain receptors in the blood vessels. You can also feel pain in the head from the surface of the scalp and from the pain receptors in the face. Pain can also be referred to the upper part of the head by dental problems. Pain from the eyes, from the neck and from the sinuses also can register as head pain or headache. If there is a change in the pressure of the cerebrospinal fluid – the liquid which helps keep the brain in place – then headaches follow. Hunting down the cause of *pain* has helped researchers produce a set of classifications of headache and it is a good way to understand what headache actually is. Recognising the *kind* of head pain you get together with other important factors like *where* it is, how often it occurs and so on can help you make a relatively quick diagnosis of what your headache is. Let's start then with the social and psychological headaches, the most commonly occurring head pains.

Mental stress headache

The main types are: muscular-contraction headache, also known as tension headache; migraine headache; and a combination of the two. There is a fourth type called 'headache of a delusional conversion' or 'hypochondriacal state' that has proved to be a bit of a mystery. It is commonly thought to arise in people with mental disturbances not caused by physical problems. Since it is likely that these people suffer from similar types of pain to other, less deluded or less hysterical people, we will treat them here as falling into one of the three other categories of psycho-social or mental headache.

30

Muscle contraction headache

This is probably the most commonly occurring of all headache. It effects both men and women and no specific age group suffers from them. They can happen at any time or to anyone. What you usually feel is a pressure in the head on both sides, rather as if someone has put a band around your forehead. Your head feels tight and the pain is dull rather than specific. You may notice it if you stand up or raise your eyes to look upwards and you realise you have been feeling uncomfortable for some time without actually registering it by moving suddenly. They seem generally to arise when you are obviously stressed or harassed and this is an important diagnostic sign. Before an exam or a job interview, after a day spent looking after the children, having to speak in public, going out on a date, asking for a raise – these are all things that you will recognise quite easily as creating the conditions for headache to arise.

What seems to happen is that you tense the muscles in your scalp, face and neck as a response to the stress you are experiencing. You don't simply frown at the thought of your boss's face, but you become tight and unrelaxed generally and when you do normal things like talking, walking and sitting your muscle groups don't have time to recover through relaxation. There is a limit to what your muscles can take and gradually the stress accumulates and is referred upwards into the head. Hence the term 'muscle-contraction' headache and hence the gradual, almost incipient onset of the pain. In contrast, blood vessel or vascular headaches, like migraine, tend to be fairly clear-cut, and this is because their action is more through the blood vessels than through the body's muscle system. As you may know, anything injected into the blood circulates much faster than if it's injected into the muscles. There is the same difference between tension headache and other forms of headache – tension headache is slow and more incipient than migraine headache and it is less widespread in the nervous system.

The pattern of pain may vary quite a lot from person to

31

person and also in the same person. It can ebb and flow during the day for example, depending on how much proper rest you take. Day to day or week to week fluctuations depend on a similar factor and, of course, on whether or not you face or can deal with your problems. A chronic mother-in-law problem has been known to cause chronic headache in sons-in-law. Remove either of the two parties and you solve the headache problem but not the fact that sons-in-law get headache.

Headache of this type can cause other damage not obviously related to the head pain. You can cause dental problems, for example, by clenching your teeth too much – especially in your sleep. Chronic headache has been known to cause suicide. Living in a state of tension isn't good for anyone and while there is little correlation between tension headache and heart illness, people with headache may be more prone to picking up minor infections that can cause discomfort.

Migraine headache
There are five major types of migraine that need concern us here but many of the symptoms in each overlap, so let's concentrate at this stage on simply understanding the nature of the differences. Most migraine attacks have certain features in common. Two thirds of migraine patients report that the pain is on one side of the head only in contrast to the muscle-contraction headache which is generally on both sides. Most migraine attacks are associated with, or preceded by, stomach and intestinal disturbances which produce nausea, vomiting or anorexia. Mood disturbances and changes in the nervous system – like numbness in the face or hands – are also often associated with the attack. We can start with the most frequently occurring type of head pain.

Common migraine. This is a severe headache of a throbbing and debilitating kind. You feel unwell, run down, on the point of bringing up and your head feels it weighs a ton. The pain can be located on one side of the head as in classical migraine but it can also occur on both sides. The attacks can go on for hours if not days. They have often been reported by women around their menstrual period but this is now thought to be a different type of migraine. What differentiates common from classical migraine is that the common form is generally less severe and does not seem to be preceded by anything like the visual and other sensory experiences common to classical migraine.

Classical migraine. This is a very painful and unpleasant syndrome that is most easily recognised by its chain of reactions. First, the person experiences a whole series of what seem quite odd sensory events. He or she often feels an air of unreality, as if they are 'not there' in some way. Though physically present, they feel mentally removed. Quite soon after this come several possible visual disturbances. Part of the visual area may be patchy or obscured by flashing lights or zig-zag patterns of light that seem to grow larger as time goes on. They also can interfere with the ability to read and this may sometimes be the person's first sense that something is wrong. Then, nausea may be felt and sometimes motor disturbances like feeling dizzy, inability to speak properly and so on. Last, but not least, is the headache. When it comes, it is usually on one side of the head, throbbing and very, very painful. Attacks almost always cripple a person for a day or two at a time and more women than men seem to suffer from them.

Cluster headache. For some time this was thought to be a separate entity from migraine but now there is growing evidence that it is a migraine variant. It consists of recurrent but relatively short-lived attacks of an intense, stabbing or boring pain felt primarily on one side of the head. At the same time there is usually a blocked nostril and red and weeping eyes. The term 'cluster' comes from the tendency of attacks to cluster together and to recur in bouts of between four and eight weeks' duration. Patients can receive between one and eight attacks a day lasting between ten minutes and two hours (Lance, 1978). People who get them also notice flushing and sweating at the same time. Males seem to suffer from this type of headache more than women, a reversal of the usually reported state of affairs.

3

Hemiplegic and ophthalmoplegic migraine. These are very much less frequently encountered than the above three categories and have fairly specific symptoms. Hemiplegic migraine is characterised by numbness or weakness felt in the hands, face or limbs before, during and after the actual head pain. Ophthalmoplegic migraine is characterised by problems associated with the muscles responsible for eye movements and so you get double vision, see a halo around normal objects and experience an inability to move the eyes properly. Again these ophthalmic symptoms may precede and follow head pain. In both cases, the headache attack itself is pretty much like a common migraine attack. The way to distinguish this type from other migraine is to note which symptoms apart from the headache are the most dominant. If you have any doubts, see your doctor. In any case, if you get this kind of migraine, see your doctor anyway – there may be other things going on inside you as well that need attention.

Basilar artery migraine. This type was only added to the classifications in 1961 when Bickerstaff published a report of his findings. Basically, this is a migraine often related to menstruation and mainly occurs in young women. The major symptoms are feelings of vertigo (inability to stand upright properly) ataxia (unsteadiness in walking) and a tendency to faint as the attack occurs. The usual signs of classical migraine are also present, including disturbances in vision and stomach and intestinal balance. Some authors have attributed the peculiar disturbances to an epileptic tendency but this has to be very carefully weighed against the fact that fainting and other motor disturbances are also associated with both shock and hysterical reactions. Young women who may have psychological problems related to their menstruation may simply collapse emotionally under both the effects of menstruation and the preliminary symptoms of migraine disturbance. We tend to forget how frightening both menstrual periods and migraine can be as separate entities to the young and uninitiated. If you get migraine during menstruation, it need not be of this type. In my experience, women who develop 'menstrual migraine' may have an initial attack of basilar artery migraine when they are in their adolescence and then settle into a pattern of common migraine.

Migraine is a widely varied phenomenon. Many people start off having one kind and then develop others or combinations of the five. In diagnosing your own problem, the important thing to remember is the central roles of both the type of headache and the related symptoms. Migraine is essentially a much bigger problem than ordinary headache, more is involved both physically and mentally, and the degree of pain and disorganisation is consequently much greater.

Combination migraine and muscle-contraction headache
Just as migraine patients tend to blend and combine the various symptoms of migraine, so it is possible for some people to have both tension headaches and migraine. If you do have both, then you probably find that you start off with a muscle-contraction headache and it gradually weaves its way into a common migraine headache attack. Some people have bouts of migraine attacks and in between develop tension headache. These can be quite clearly recognised for what they are.

That concludes the section on the first level of headaches. What marks them off from the second level that we are about to describe is the fact that, in general, mental and social stress headache has a routine and well-developed pattern that is clearly recognised as stress-induced. The following headache usually has a clear and well-defined physical or medical base.

Mild to moderate risk physical headache
The best way to describe this kind of headache is to make a distinction between benign headache – that is, headache that has a physical or organic cause – and malignant headache – headache that can cause serious, even fatal, physical stress. For example, it is possible to get a headache from a sinus infection. A *benign* sinus headache may disappear fairly quickly

as the infection disappears. However, the same symptom, headache, may have a *malignant* base as, for example, in *nasopharyngeal carcinoma*, found commonly in China and South East Asia, which is far more serious and involves destruction of the nerves in the nasal region. Cough headache – the head pain that some people get when they cough – may have both a benign or malignant base. You may be simply irritating a sinus condition or a low-grade tension headache, or you may be disturbing a tumour. In this chapter, we will concentrate on benign bases but remember that the same symptom (headache) can be common to both states. Read the rest of this chapter in close conjunction with the next one.

Food and drink
Various foods, as we noted earlier, can give you headaches and these are generally benign. Some people have a resistance to the monosodium glutamate which is used excessively in the preparation of Chinese meals as well as being used in cured meat foods like hot dogs. It is the concentration of nitrite used in the colouring process of the meat that does the trick. Recent studies, however, have not been able to pinpoint precisely what it is that does the damage. It is now, for instance, thought that monosodium glutamate may not be the chemical agent involved in Chinese food. Either way, these aren't very serious instances. If you eat ripe cheeses or drink red wine while taking a Monoamine oxidase inhibitor (MAO) drug for psychiatric disturbance, the result may not be so pleasant. There have even been cases of death reported (Blackwell, 1963). So if you are on drugs like parnate, nardil or marplan, be careful. The cheese *et al* increase your blood pressure rapidly and give you a sudden headache. I was once called to attend to one such sufferer who had been warned by her doctor to stay off cheese but didn't – there is very little medicine can do for this headache – and I had to watch a very distressed lady go through two days of hell before the effects wore off. The drugs, by the way, are used in the treatment of depression, anxiety and, in some cases, psychosis.

If you like ice-cream, why not indulge yourself? But if it gives you a headache, it is usually due to pain being referred from the palate or the throat, caused in turn by the drop in temperature of the mouth or pharynx. If you suffer from migraine this may be all you need to set off an attack. The migraine mechanism seems remarkably indiscriminate – it goes off for no reason at all sometimes.

Drinking can precipitate migraine attacks in some people. Ethyl alcohol makes the arteries in the head swell, hence the pain and the trigger-ability of drinking. But it doesn't *cause* headache or migraine in everybody, nor in many people who suffer from migraine as a routine. This leads one to suppose that either those who do have attacks when they drink are especially susceptible to ethyl alcohol or that drinking has become psychologically linked to migraine or headache – inducing mechanisms in the individual. Of course drinking to excess can cause most people to have a hangover headache the next day and certain types of alcoholic beverages seem to have a particular ability – if taken in large enough quantities – to give you a headache. Rough brandies are one such example but, again, this also depends on your physical and emotional state. If you're run down or keyed up, or both, you may be more prone to the effects of alcohol than at other times.

Coffee drinkers, beware – deciding to stop drinking the stuff abruptly can give you a headache from caffeine withdrawal, so try and reduce your 'fix' slowly and carefully.

Headaches from hobbies

This is a broad category and you'll see why in just a moment. People who enjoy swimming in winter may get a headache from the sudden exposure to cold water. Likewise, avid walkers or joggers may get a headache from a cold wind or going out in very cold weather. Headaches arising in both activities are worsened by dental problems. Wearing a sweatband while running or playing a sport may also give you a headache. Some adolescent school children report getting headache while playing games. In the benign form this is not very serious but for migraine sufferers it can be quite debilitating. This form of 'exertional' headache can, however, have a more serious or malignant side. In rare instances it could be the first indication of a malignant growth or of structural damage in the brain. For details, see the next chapter.

Mountain climbers, especially those who go above 10,000 feet may suffer from acute mountain sickness which first registers itself as a form of tension headache of unpleasant intensity. Any sport or hobby which involves long periods of intense concentration – such as watching football on television – can cause headache through a mixture of emotional deprivation (anger and distress caused by an own-goal or your team losing), muscle tension and keeping the spine immobile for too long. Of course, excessive drinking and smoking at the same time contribute to their share of the damage.

Sexual intercourse – I told you this was a very broad category – can surprisingly cause headache. Lance (1978) identifies three kinds – those occurring as a result of muscle contraction as the level of excitement mounts, those occurring unfortunately at or about orgasm (due to blood pressure increase) and a third kind which becomes worse on standing up and seems due to a torn membrane between the brain and spinal cord. None of them seem to be too serious a matter but if they persist, you should see a doctor.

Headache from illness

At the simplest and most obvious level, you get headache from blows to the head, from concussion after accidents and, sometimes, from having an operation. None of these need be malignant. You also can get a headache some months *after* a trauma and that needs a little more careful assessment (see next chapter).

Fevers of any kind give you a headache and often mark the onset of an infectious illness, due to the swelling of the brain arteries. It gets more intense as the fever progresses, especially in typhoid, tularemia, polio, malaria, trichinosis, infectious mononuclueosis and ordinary 'flu. Sometimes you get a headache from medical probes. Lumbar punctures, angio grams, even EEGs* have been known to give quite benign headache (benign but painful, that is – they disappear after a few hours or days or weeks, depending on the glibness of your doctor). I have known patients who have developed migraine simply at the thought of going to see a doctor. For some strange reason, this applies even more about going to see dentists!

Sinusitis, as we have said, along with dental problems – especially from caries or root infections – can cause unpleasant pulsating headache that is made worse by any movement, blowing the nose, leaning forward, bending down, as well as by exposure to cold temperatures, water and wind. Sometimes your teeth may not bite properly due to inattention or poor dental treatment and you can get a headache owing to the imbalance in the muscle stress. If you feel lopsided when you eat *and* you get headache, do have your teeth seen to first. It's a fairly straightforward procedure, well worth the trouble and (or) the accompanying fear-induced migraine.

Your eyes can give you a benign muscle-based headache due to strain, weakness in focusing or light sensitivity. The eye disease *glaucoma* can cause pain expressed deep inside the eye which spreads over the forehead. This must be seen to, as must any eye disturbance associated with headache that causes peculiarities in vision, whether blurring, double-vision, mistiness or haloes around lights.

Problems and diseases associated with the neck and spine can also cause headache and again should be seen by a doctor when they occur. Sometimes sleeping in a particularly uncomfortable position can cause you a back or neck ache which on its own doesn't cause headache. If you then try to limp or otherwise minimise the strain, you may give yourself a headache by putting too much pressure on your neck and head-support muscles as you tend to favour one side or the other.

* EEGs are the recordings made of the brain's electrical activity. Lumbar punctures are used to determine the pressure and state of the cerebro-spinal fluid. They generally involve removing quantities of the fluid from an area in the spine.

The trick is *not* to overcompensate. Your muscles will recover on their own provided you rest them.

There are certain medical illnesses that are not obviously linked to headache and of which headache is not a diagnostic symptom, which nevertheless do cause headache sometimes. Mild cases of hypertension (basically, high blood pressure) for example, can give occasional headaches and severe sufferers can have them more often – usually on waking from their sleep. Sometimes lack of sleep itself, perhaps through illness or emotional stress, can cause a headache.

If you don't eat properly, headaches may occur. Missing a meal in normal people can sometimes have the same effect.

Hyperthyroidism, hypothyroidism, hypoparathyroidism and hypoadrenal function may all produce headache and, to continue this series of 'h's', hypoglycaemia can also have headache as one of its accompanying symptoms, as too can hyperinsulinism in diabetic sufferers. See your doctor and he or she will help.

In addition to all this there are some people who, for one reason or another, experience odd pains and twinges on the head, scalp and face. These may be malignant but often they are not and may be caused by nothing more serious than sleeping in an awkward position, wearing a new hairstyle or jarring your skull. The important thing is to look for a pattern and to notice any sign of a worsening or spreading in incidence. Act immediately and you could save yourself a lot of trouble. It could be that an old injury or scar has started work again or it could be that you are upset and need psychological help. Neither should be neglected.

CHAPTER FIVE

When are headaches dangerous?

So far so good. What we have described as psychological head-ache and benign physical headache (if you can call malaria benign) are fairly clearly recognised and dealt with. What, though, about headache that can be dangerous, cause serious, irreversible damage, perhaps even death? How do you tell the difference between a benign and a malignant headache and how long should you let a headache trouble you before you get help? After all, since so many headaches are psychological in origin, it is natural to assume that any headache that troubles you is probably due to tension and will go away in time. Certainly, if everyone took every headache they got to a doctor, there is a distinct possibility that the medical profession would collapse under the strain.

The problem is that it can be very difficult for even a trained professional to accurately differentiate between a benign and malignant headache on simple examination – even, sometimes, after thorough examination. Worse, ordinary headache like migraine can in extreme cases cause brain damage or deteriora-tion. So what I have to say in this chapter has to be treated fairly cautiously. At best, it is a rough guide, always to be used in conjunction with your doctor.

To start with, let's deal with what we know best. Some people have been known to kill themselves after many years of suffering from chronic headache without relief. The notion that headache can drive you mad may not be strictly accurate but the incidence of suicide in headache sufferers who are not treated successfully, for whom no drug or type of psychotherapy works, is high (Simons, 1969). Which only goes to show just how far headache can drive you. Imagine what it is like to go to sleep with a headache, wake up with one and carry one around with you all day, every day, for years and years. This is one form of dangerous headache.

Migraine can cause problems that are worrying. Basilar artery migraine sufferers, because of their proneness to temporal losses of consciousness, can place their lives in jeopardy and there have been some reports of heart disorders associated with the condition (Petersen *et al*, 1977). Breathing failure in hemiplegic migraine has also been reported (Neligan *et al*, 1977). Both these instances can cause serious damage to the heart but both are relatively rare. Rare, too, is death from migraine attack (and hard to establish) but there have been cases reported in medical literature. Prolonged and excessive occurrences of migraine over many years seem to cause a slight but cumulative level of damage while single attacks on their own don't have much organic effect (Hungerford *et al*, 1976). Migraine has been linked to persisting *hemiparesis* (muscular weakness), *ophthalmoplegic* and visual field defects, brain *infarcts* (areas of dead tissue caused by a blocked artery) and facial weaknesses, all of which can be permanent. More clear-cut evidence for damage may in time be forthcoming now that researchers have access to brain scanners, like the EMI scanner, called computerised axial tomographs or CATs but it is early days yet for this new source of data.

The silver lining to this dark cloud is that if you do have chronic headache or are a known headache sufferer, having had your headache examined by a doctor at one time or another, the chances of your developing or having a *dangerous* headache are fairly small – especially if you have suffered for five years or more. The really clear-cut worrying sign is if you have a sudden acute headache when you least expect it or if you don't usually get headache and you get a sudden, intense one. Some people who are headache sufferers periodically may also get one for no accountable reason. Most people who have regular headache will know their own patterns and it is the acute headache out of pattern that may be a danger. Now, what causes these?

Firstly, of course, you may have a simple fever as we remarked in Chapter Four. More severe fevers or fevers left unattended may cause far more intense symptoms. If you have a stiff neck with your headache, if you find you can't stand light, bright or otherwise, and you have a temperature, do something about it quickly. If, in addition, or in fact at any time, you get a kind of creeping drowsiness *and* a headache, see a doctor. If the pupil of one eye is significantly larger than the other, if you have numbness or a paralysing feeling on one side (or both), see a doctor.

The reasons for these symptoms may be benign but they may also be malignant. Space-occupying impairments in the brain, for example, tend to cause sudden headache and drowsiness when you are *not* usually drowsy. Bleeding from angiomas (a form of non-malignant tumour) in the brain can cause headache and neck stiffness followed in a few hours or days by pains in the back, buttocks and thighs. Another sign of trouble is nausea or vomiting with a sudden headache and you don't suffer from migraine.

At the other end of the scale, there are certain symptoms that leave – or should leave – you and those around you in no doubt that the headache is dangerous. Sudden acute headache followed by loss of consciousness, no matter how many hours later, is likely to be caused by a brain haemorrhage which you may or may not survive. Some of the people who have survived reported that it feels as if something suddenly gives way in the brain. The head pain starts, incidentally, on one side and quite rapidly spreads over the head to the back and into the neck. Headache with difficulty in standing, balancing or walking (I don't mean just dizziness or hysterical dizziness where you put on a show for sympathy or attention, I mean when you really can't stand up properly and tend to fall over, or if you begin to walk funnily), usually means a muscle-control co-ordination disturbance, definitely to be attended to.

43

Drowsiness again, with *confusion, disorientation* and the inevitable headache, less acute in onset though, may mean that you have meningitis, encephalitis or some other diffuse infection of the brain. You may experience difficulty in placing your chin against your chest and find that the attempt to do so increases the head pain considerably. Be careful, though, because some psychiatric drugs, especially certain phenothiazines and especially if used in large quantities and in conjunction with other drugs to reduce the side-effects of the first drug (!) – have precisely the same effect. See whoever prescribed the drugs *first* and you could save yourself a lot of trouble.

If you have a headache and you feel that your body (not just your head, we all think our heads are huge when we have a headache) is larger or smaller than it really is, if you can't understand words, can't talk or read properly (not, of course, if you usually get classical migraine), can't distinguish left from right or carry out things you could do the day before, you need help. There may be some damage in one or other of your brain hemispheres. Of course, you may have also just suffered a huge emotional shock – so use your common sense in diagnosing which it is.

Talking of common sense, check your sense of smell. If you have a cold or sinusitis or your nose is blocked, you won't smell much, but if you have a headache without nose blocking *and* no sense of smell, you could have damaged a nerve or have a tumour blocking your sense receiving pathways. If, in addition to no sense of smell, your intellect seems impaired (don't just ask your wife or husband to help you assess this – they may be biased) and you get confused, you could have a tumour in the front region of your head that is causing all the trouble.

Pregnancy tends to cure headache, especially migraine. If you get a headache during your pregnancy, tread carefully – it could be the first signs of poison in your blood. Call in outside help quickly.

Sudden intense pain behind one eye, which may move upwards so that it seems like a headache as well, may be caused

44

by changing aneurysm (swelling in the walls of blood vessels) in the brain. Attend to it right away because it may also be the eye disease glaucoma. Pain in the ear – especially acute pain – and headache have been obvious signs of serious problems since Hippocrates' time, so don't ignore them. You could have a thrombosis in your sinuses or be developing an abscess on your brain.

These then are the extremes. The problem we all face, doctors and laymen alike, is that somewhere in between lies a whole series of headaches that are really tough to diagnose properly, sometimes with tragic and unintentional results. I know of one man who went to see his doctor, concerned about a sudden headache such as we have just described and was offered an EEG (electroencephelogram, see page 39) to re-assure him that there was nothing wrong. So worried was the man that his well-intentioned doctor had suggested an EEG, he drove himself into a state of panic during which he suffered a fatal heart attack. On post-mortem, there was no sign of brain damage or disturbance other than that caused by the heart attack. In another case, a woman who suffered from migraine refused consistently to have a skull X-ray and brain scan requested by her doctor who had become concerned about her drastic weight loss. Her argument was that her feeling poorly, her weight loss and her headache were all caused by migraine – so why go to the trouble, the pain and the expense of having the investigations done? She died a few months later from a brain tumour. Tragically and paradoxically, she was partly right. The headache she had suffered periodically for thirty years had not been caused by the tumour – the migraine had been responsible for that – but the headache in her last months had. Her tumour had grown to quite a size *before* it began to press on areas that cause headache. As I said earlier, the brain is not sensitive to internal pain, it is only when something registers on the edges that pain is felt.

I don't believe that anything can be gained by hiding these problems from the general public and pretending that we can diagnose head conditions more accurately than we really can.

Technology helps, of course, and we would be lost were it not for the modern advances in radiology, investigative surgery and behaviour assessment. But far more can be achieved if you, the reader, realise the limitations of the technologies we employ. A brain X-ray, for example, is just what it says it is – a simple photograph of the brain, not a cross-section or a detailed examination of each aspect of the brain. If you take a photograph in a dark room, you get a black picture. What you need is light to help you see. The same applies in X-rays of the brain, so coloured dyes are injected into the arteries to bring light, as it were, to the mass of the brain. If parts of the brain are obscured by other parts then you can't see them and you have to guess what has happened. This is where problems of diagnosis occur.

'Surely,' you might ask, 'there are tests, behavioural or psychological tests, to help tell precisely what a head pain means. Surely there are certain patterns of behaviour associated with dangerous headache?'

Well, yes, there are. But only in certain cases. There are tests for brain damage, for example, which can pick up extreme and, in some cases, moderate, impairments in ability, but to interpret these impairments is another problem altogether. People with severe brain damage, for example, show deterioration in their intellect and movements but so too do some elderly people who are not seriously brain damaged, schizophrenics, depressives, hysterics and a whole variety of other people with mental or emotional disturbances. When it comes to assessing moderate to mild damage, the problem naturally escalates. Even perfectly normal people have wide fluctuations in their behaviours and abilities, making comparative assessment very difficult, especially if you are looking for the dangerous needle in the benign headache haystack.

So, what can you do to help at this level? First, you can get to know yourself better, to help both you and/or your doctor. Pay attention to things instead of brushing them aside. If you have a numbness, for example, or a funny feeling in your neck or back or head, or your bones and joints seem to ache, find out why. Don't leave it, hoping it will go away. It may very well do so, but find out just in case. Learn to open your mouth about yourself. In my opinion too many people suffer in silence. They put up with quite startling levels of pain and discomfort without a murmur. Other people insist on treating themselves, quite unaware of the damage they may do in the process. This applies especially to headache where people tend to take painkillers as if they were disappearing from the shelves. Damage to the basic systems of the body, such as the liver, can follow and certain painkillers can even cause headache themselves. Worse, you could be treating yourself for what you think is an ordinary headache and employ painkillers that obscure other symptoms that may otherwise alert you to the fact that you could have a dangerous headache. Moreover, you and your packet of aspirin or unprescribed tranquillisers could also be confusing your doctor. One slow-developing symptom of certain brain problems, for example, is a kind of nerve deafness, where over a length of time you gradually lose your senses of perception which become slowly but surely deadened. Pain killers taken for headache can obscure this.

Secondly, use your common sense. Think things out before you see a doctor so that you can give him or her the information he or she needs to know accurately and can volunteer stuff she or he may miss. A bump on the head that you thought was nothing – in fact, you may have forgotten about it – may be causing your headache now, even if you got the bump weeks ago. Head pains from bangs on the head aren't all just simple concussion. You could have more serious damage. Similarly, old illnesses – such infections as meningitis, encephalitis, TB, operations that you thought were over and done with – can have complications or even recur, causing headache.

Certain medicines can reactivate some old scar sites, so be sure to have this information recorded somewhere – don't just rely on your doctor. If you had an illness, an operation or a bang on the head or are taking medicines prescribed by another doctor, write it all down in your diary. In this age of movement and pressure, people go overseas, have accidents in other towns, infections in foreign countries, move job, move country, take drugs here and there (not all countries have the same regulations about drugs – I have known people buy a drug in Europe, for example, that contains elements not found in the same drug made and bought in London), see psychiatrists they are too emabarrassed to tell their doctors about – and get second and secret opinions that they are equally embarrassed about. All these can in their own way contribute to giving you a headache or perhaps even obscure the presence of a dangerous one. *You* have to take some responsibility for your body. You only have the one.

Thirdly, get to know your body and its functions. Examine yourself, feel your head. Run your hand through your hair and feel your scalp and get used to the pattern of your skull. Have a look at your veins, find out where the major arteries are. Don't panic though – your head has quite a few odd-feeling lumps and things as well as a few areas that are always sensitive to pain. Get your doctor to show you where they are. Certain scalp infections can cause a kind of head pain. Scratching your head excessively can also irritate both your scalp and your muscular system. Watch for swellings and indentations. Feel your veins and arteries and look for hardening or tenderness – especially if you're getting on in years. Your headache may be related to arteries in your temples. Tap your head every once in a while and see if it hurts. *Tap*, I said. And not when you've got a headache or sinusitus.

Do you have trouble chewing, or pain when you talk that you can't quite pin down to a particular area or cause? The arteries around your skull may be narrowing for some reason worth discovering. If you knew yourself well, you would be able to distinguish between that and tension-induced jaw, mouth and head pain.

Keep an eye on your skin and your general physical condition. Severe weight loss for no obvious reason with headache is cause to worry. If your skin gets noticeably smoother, paler, waxen and dry, or there is a change in the growth rate of your body hair, with headache, you could have a deficiency in your

48

pituitary gland at the base of your brain which controls, among other things, the secretion of body hormones. Headache and impotence in sexual performance may be the results of a passing emotional trauma but they could be caused by damage to a lobe in the temples. Keeping in touch with your general level of symptoms could help your doctor make a quick and, for you, very relieving diagnosis.

Fourthly, learn to recognise that, as you get older, you are going to get more prone to certain kinds of physical problems – including headache – that don't effect you when you are younger. You can get headache after shingles (*herpetic* infection), for example, something that usually affects middle- to old-aged people. And, of course, advancing age brings with it a general and depressing deterioration in the level and capacity of bodily functions, one symptom of which could be headache.

Lastly, don't forget your children. They get headache for a number of reasons, some of which are serious. Any headache in association with earache must be checked on as must headache that follows ear infections or bad coughs and colds. Polio and other similar illnesses, although far less common nowadays, also cause headache. Watch out for headache and stiff necks, drowsiness and so on, in your children. Like adults, they could have contracted a potentially dangerous infection. Have chronic sinus conditions *very carefully* assessed, even if it means taking a second or third opinion. I have known parents and doctors expose children to the most traumatic of treatment régimes, including extensive surgery, simply to cure (rather, *not* always to cure) headache arising out of a sinus condition, or adenoids or hay fever, conditions which may have responded to a little warmth and affection given to the child, or insight given to the parents. The possible benefits of these procedures has to be weighed against the damage they do to the child's psychological make up.

An important condition to look for in children is epilepsy and to distinguish it from migraine attacks or early acute confusional migraine (Ehyia and Fenichel, 1978. See Chapter 8). Here's a brief check list to help you sort out what is what:

1. Children who get migraine as they get older often get stomach and intestinal disturbances, including vomiting attacks associated with headache, before full and proper attacks develop. They also suffer from car sickness. Not so in epileptic children.

2. In epileptic children, the headache is quite brief, usually lasting less than ten minutes. It comes on suddenly and severely. Migraine headaches in children last longer and come on more slowly.

3. The epileptic child's headache is often followed by drowsiness, a stupor of varying degrees of confusion and, in many cases, disturbances in consciousness. Not so in migraine, although it is easy to mistake a depressed, upset and heavily slumped child for a drowsy and stuperous one. Either way, see a doctor.

4. The real difference comes out, though, in the reactions of the different illnesses to drug treatments. Migraine medication (see Chapter 9) has no effect on epileptic headache.

Personally, I think that if your child gets headache – especially if he or she is under twelve – you should regard it as potentially dangerous, irrespective of whether or not it is physically dangerous. Having your doctor check it causes no harm and, more important, having *you* attend to it can help your child enormously. Like animals, children have very little real ability or the necessary rights or facilities to express themselves. Many children resort to physical illness, particularly headache, to make themselves heard. Children are children, not to be confused with little adults. A headache for a child is, I believe, a far more significant and massive psychological statement than it is for an adult. For some of them, it's all they've got. It may also be why so many children grow up to be headache sufferers as adults – which takes us right back to square one, doesn't it?

CHAPTER SIX

What causes headache?

Now that the descriptive aspect of the book is done with, we can go on to have a look at the causes of headache to see the deeper reasons behind headache and to get the relative importance of the various kinds of headache into perspective. One of the reasons why headaches have caused so much confusion in the past is because there hasn't been a proper overall view. Headache, as you will now probably appreciate, can be caused by a pretty wide range of things and not by a single factor. Yet many people have attempted to lump all headache under a single label. We won't be doing that here. There are different types of headache; some are common, some are rare. In the next two chapters, we will try to give you some idea of what causes what and the agents that seem to be responsible for each type of headache. We will focus in Chapter 7 on psychological causes of headache, but first we will look at physical ones.

To begin with, I want to introduce an idea to help you understand why it is that we can't say there is *one* basic cause of headache. In medicine, as indeed in all sciences, we have to distinguish between simple and complex causes of events. If you get a broken arm or leg, the cause is simple – you fell out of a tree, off the roof or something hit your arm. However, the cause and effect chain is only that simple *provided* we absolutely and rigidly refuse to examine events any further. In the early days of medicine, this was a commonplace procedure and you got a neat blend of witchcraft, quackery and vivid imaginationitis. Medical events were 'explained' – and, worse, treated – by a whole range of irrelevant procedures, just because they happened to occur *before* the injury. Elements of this method of approach are still to be found in some quarters. As recently as 1967, for example, I heard of a doctor, well-qualified and experienced, who prescribed a glass of water for the removal of warts. I was unable to discover whether you had to say the spell before or after drinking the water.

Nothing in either medicine or nature is simple. We only *choose* to make it simple. What makes them complicated is the fact that everything is intricately related to everything else in ways that have to be explored in each and every instance – just in case we, the scientists or doctors, have missed something. Often major breakthroughs in medicine have been made by a dedicated researcher acting on a hunch and examining a link that his or her colleagues had dismissed as irrelevant or insignificant.

Let's go back to our broken arm example. Now *you're* a doctor and someone calls you to attend a broken arm. If you believe in simple cause and effect, you will treat the fracture, patch up the arm and leave it. The patient fell and the fall broke his or her arm. How would you feel, though, if a week later, the patient fell again and again broke his arm? And again the week after that? It can happen. Would you still feel happy with your simple view of cause and effect? I think not. You could be dealing with an arm-breaking freak who likes pain (unlikely), a terribly accident-prone person (not so unlikely) or disturbance in the brain that is affecting your patient's balance (rare, but possible). You *need* a complex-based theory of cause and effect to make sure that an apparently simple matter really is straightforward. Further, *simple* things like broken arms happen to *complex* things like people. How a person *reacts* to the break, how they help cause it – in a medical and psychological sense – are very important in understanding why these things happen.

Modern medicine is slowly but surely modifying its theory of disease to encompass the need to have a more complex parallel theory of cause. Until quite recently it was thought that diseases were caused fundamentally by external factors –

infections, germs, traumatic events and so on – invading the essentially sound and antiseptic body. Getting rid of the foreign invasion, it was thought, restored the body to normal, an idea that is only partially true. Some diseases do operate like this but the *total* picture is much more complex. Take the common cold. Ostensibly, you catch a 'cold' germ and as the upper-respiratory tract infection sets in you start to feel miserable. But why do you get a cold at some times and not others? Cold germs are around (if they exist in such simple form) most of the time. The answer probably lies in the fact that, sitting in draughts apart, there is a complex relationship between your level of resistance to respiratory tract infections and your general psychological and emotional state, your level of fatigue and bodily condition, your propensity to smoke or drink, etc, etc, etc . . .

When you get to more complicated illnesses that involve the whole body or, more important, the higher functions of nerve activity, things can become incredibly confusing. Cancer, for example, is a real problem for just this kind of reason. At the risk of offending cancer researchers, I will say that head pain falls into the same category.

The head is, after the heart, the single most important unit of the body. Without it (!), everything else ceases. The brain is the body's headquarters; it organises and regulates much of the activity of the rest of the body. More important still is the fact that the head is the source of consciousness and through this our experience of and contact with the entire psychological and social world around us.

This makes at least three possible sources of headache: disturbance from the environment, disturbance from the body itself, either through injury or illness, and disturbance from within its own structures. Each of these can arise at the same time and interact with the others. So, now let's examine causes of headache from this complex perspective and try to make some (common) sense out of the mass of ideas about causes that already exist in the medical and public minds.

The mechanisms of head pain

Earlier on, I said that most pain is registered primarily at the sites of entry and exit of the brain's blood supply. I mentioned, too, that changes in the pressure of the *cerebrospinal* fluid – fluid that effects the nervous system via the brain and spine – can also cause head pain.* Let's go on from there. We know we have a headache when we have pain in the pain pickup points in the head. So what happens to cause the pain? At the simplest level, pain is caused by anything that interferes with the blood flow to and from the brain, either through an increased pressure of blood which makes the vessels expand or swell, or through inflammation and blockage. The nerves that transmit the onset of pain are connected up through branches and tributaries and linked with the pain-feeling nerves on the face and scalp and in the muscles of the head and neck. Pain can then be referred to other sites of the head, depending on the level and organisation of the nervous systems involved.

So what we have to consider to understand head pain are: what constituents in the blood can cause changes in the structure of the arteries and veins and make them inflamed? What can squeeze or pinch the blood vessels to cause pain to register? What can block them or push them aside – thus causing pain through stretching them? What can increase blood pressure to make them painful? And what can refer pain through the nerve network so that the head itself appears to ache?

Some of the answers to these questions have already been given. We have talked about pain transmitted from the roots of the teeth, from earache and eye-ache and from the sinus conditions. We have also discussed things like the phenomena of muscle-contraction which causes headache without interfering directly with the flow of blood in the major arteries. These are fairly clearly understandable, as too, you will appreciate, is the idea of disease or malfunction in the nerves' transmission of pain. *Tic douloureux*, or *trigeminal neuralgia*, for example, is a disorder of one of the major nerve pathways of the brain,

* Strictly speaking we should also include muscular tension in this list but the blood-flow cause is a very convenient example to work with.

54

involving the *trigeminal* nerve and its roots which transmit pain information from the front two thirds of the head. It feels a lot like cluster headache, having a pain pattern of short, jabbing intensity with recurring bouts in clusters. But it starts in the cheek or chin, gets worse as you get older and does not appear to involve the blood vessel flow. Ice-cream headache also affects the *trigeminal* nerve but not dangerously so. It simply overstimulates it. The same nerve system, though, can be affected by tumours or swellings on or near it and their action is similar to those described further on.

What must concern us more, however, are the causes of the brain's blood flow disturbance. By examining how this disturbance operates, we can make some of the descriptions given in Chapters 4 and 5 understandable. It will be convenient to start with the simple, more clearly physical causes and then look at the more complex ones.

First, an artery or vein can be interfered with by traction, that is, movement of parts of the brain. When you have, for example, a lumbar puncture to investigate the state of your *cerebrospinal* fluid, the entry of the needle in your back to sample the fluid lowers the pressure of the fluid, causing the brain to pull against its supports. This traction literally pulls or jars the blood vessels and you get a headache at the site of this jarring – that is, in the head. When you have a tumour, a similar thing happens, only this time, instead of the brain pulling on its supports, the tumour within the brain pushes, as it grows, against other masses. This *traction* causes the blood vessels to be pulled or pushed aside out of their normal orbits. If lesions, such as tumours, abscesses or haematomas, are strategically sited on or near blood supply roots, they can swell and block or pinch the vessels as well. All result in a headache. Any kind of head injury – a blow to the head, a whiplash injury or, less seriously, the effects of sudden halt, as in a car – cause headache through movement of the brain and brain vessels. Like a bruise on the arm which swells outwards, a bruise in the brain swells and pushes other organs out of place.

You could also be born with an actual malfunction of the blood vessels which only comes to light as you grow older. The severity of the problem naturally varies with the degree of malfunction: fits and comas may be induced as too will headache. Also, anything that increases the pressure in the brain, such as blockages in the *cerebrospinal* fluid pathways and a range of other possibilities, can cause pain to be registered.

Secondly, infections like fevers, *encephalitis* or *meningitis*, can cause inflammation of the blood vessels which stimulates the pain receivers. Where and when determines the level of headache and variety of other symptoms presented.

Moving on to more complex causes of irritation of the blood vessels, some substances carried in the blood can cause painful swelling in the vessels, particularly substances that regulate the blood flow, chemical in poisons and in some foods. We have already talked about food and poisons in earlier chapters. The complexity arises, however, because while such things in the blood as *histamine* and *Bradykinin* and certain poisons *always* cause head pain, certain others – especially food substances – do not. Sometimes the same person can eat the same food on separate occasions and get a headache on one occasion but not on the other. Further, isolating the headache-making substance does not necessarily help a great deal in establishing a headache trigger. Often, only some people seem to be prone to the substance, but why this is so is not altogether clear. It may be something that is inherited and it may not. We will look at this aspect in the next chapter. The headache induced by MAO inhibitors and certain foods occurs because of the rapid increase in blood pressure brought about by the interaction between the drug and chemicals in certain foods. High blood pressure alone, however, does not necessarily cause headache.

Higher order mechanisms in headache formation
So long as we stay at the level of simple cause and effect, things like the above are easy to understand. When we start considering the brain as a complex whole and its relation to its

blood vessels, nerve and muscular systems, it becomes more difficult to understand. Add to that the idea of the whole organism continually reacting with its environment and, to coin a phrase, one's head begins to ache. It is into this category that the vast majority of headaches fall and so it is the most important part of the book. What we need to do here is set the overall picture to prepare us for the next chapter.

Take the basic idea we have been using so far – the notion that disturbances in the brain's blood vessels cause headache. Now consider it in terms of a normal, healthy individual. Assume that there is absolutely nothing wrong with you, no tumours, no inherited malfunction in blood flow, no infections, no allergies to foods – nothing. Technically, and leaving aside muscle-tension headache, you should be headache-free, right?

Wrong. The blood vessel system, even if functioning perfectly, is open to misuse because it is controlled and operated by centres high up in the central nervous system or, if you prefer, by the mind.

The way to understand this is to imagine that an absolute idiot is given a beautifully engineered, totally efficient, brand new motor car. Under normal circumstances, one would expect it to last for at least a year. But if our idiot insists on constantly sending the rev counter into red on every gear change, including reverse, refuses to add oil or water or charge the battery, stops the car by throwing it into reverse, insists on cornering on two wheels and using the car like a jeep – then it won't last very long. This, very roughly, is what happens to the human brain in the hands of some people and it may be why headaches and migraines occur. Let us briefly, therefore, look at some of the ways in which the higher nervous system controls the phenomena of head pain.

For a start, the control of the brain's blood vessels lies in the hands of the *autonomic* nervous system. This is the system that regulates the entire body's level of activity, and it is subdivided into the *sympathetic sub-system*, which is responsible for co-ordinating the arousal of all the body's systems and the *para-sympathetic system* which relaxes them or puts them

57

down after activity. Simply put, the *sympathetic* system arouses the body and its systems in times of stress, excitement and so on, while the *para-sympathetic* system calms it down and returns it to normal. In addition to this, the walls of the arteries have muscle cells which operate partly independently of the *autonomic* nervous system to regulate the blood pressure of the blood flow as it enters the brain. If blood pressure drops it swells and if it rises it narrows. This system operates under normal conditions irrespective of the individual moderate ups and downs of bodily activity.

However, it ceases to function during certain emergencies, of which migraine attacks are one. This has led us to suppose that its function may be overridden by higher centres. Much the same may apply to the pattern of *autonomic* nervous system activities. Over-arousal or prolonged arousal without a corresponding period of relaxation may overstress or over-extend the sympathetic nervous system. It can also throw the two sub-systems out of synchronisation so that relaxation may not occur when the level of over-arousal is finally reduced. This is rather like the way tension headache occurs. Further, the two systems may not have fully developed in some adults and not all the systems get aroused in unison. Components of the sub-systems may also operate in conflict or confusion. In a simple sense you can compare the way they control and regulate the action of the brain's blood vessels to our idiot driver stopping and starting the perfectly efficient car.

As you will appreciate, we have entered a grey area in medical research. We don't know a great deal about how the various levels of higher brain activity perform and much is still interesting theory, untested and, in some cases, untried. The *autonomic* nervous system is intricately connected with many major brain systems including those areas of the brain that are regarded as the seat of the emotions – the *limbic* system, the *hypothalamus*, *thalamus*, the hormone-secreting *pituitary* and so on. To take one example: pituitary control of hormones may have some influence on the development of headache as we have seen but psychological changes in the individual may be responsible for the pituitary receiving orders to secrete to a certain pattern in the first place. Hormonal secretions from the pituitary may cause a headache disturbance at one time but not at another simply because the individual is in a state of arousal or excitement at one time but not another – as, for example, during a monthly period. Like the migraine attack's effect on the *autogenic* muscle activity in the artery wall, the arousal may override the hormonal influences.

The point is that the relationships between the various higher order systems are complex and remain a puzzle. What we must do is to accept this and recognise it without running away from the problem in order to seek simple solutions. In the following chapters, we will try to come to grips with some of the complexity involved in order to help you help yourself. Stay loose.

Last word on simple causes

The simple and straightforward causes of headache, like brain tumour, account for a very low number of all recorded headache. There is also a low incidence of headaches from eating the wrong food or from a poor diet, despite many popular views. Pearce (1975), for example, found them to occur in only 13 per cent of people in his migraine study, so they are a comparatively minor cause in the general population overall. Headache from poisons, from industrial chemicals and other substances occurs with more frequency but only in those industries where the individual is exposed to risk (like the possibility of Q fever in abattoir workers) so this need not concern the average person. Travel and altitude headaches are other fairly clear-cut cause-effect types.

You can get headache when you experience physical problems, such as having a period, high blood pressure, from exposure to extreme sound or light or even from constipation. But there is considerable doubt whether each on its own actually creates an effect on the blood vessels of the brain. Worry or over-tension about blood pressure, constipation, periods and the like, are more likely to give you a headache than the actual problem itself. Extreme noise can be painful in the ears but how you react emotionally and the level of your stimulator and relaxer functions is the thing that causes the pain in the head. Likewise light exposure.

You may be free from headache during pregnancy, after emptying your bowels, lowering your blood pressure or avoiding extremes of sound and light, but this does not show how the headache is actually caused. It may be that you stop being tense or anxious or that you have learnt to associate headache-producing internal cues with certain trigger stimuli and feel quite safe in their absence. The best way to think about them is to consider them as important *parts* of your headache syndrome and go on from there to a full and complex analysis of the cause.

CHAPTER SEVEN

Headache as a psychosomatic problem

To say that headache is a psychosomatic problem is to say what? In the heyday of simple psychosomatics (only recently ended) it meant that your physical problem was caused by your psychological state. Learned and unlearned people alike went around solemnly pronouncing that literally every illness was psychological. I once made a list of all the things I had read that were supposedly caused by the mind. Everything from cancer to heart disease found its way on to that list.

Now things have changed. The vogue thing these days is biochemistry; everything is caused by chemicals. We now talk about biorhythms, neurochemistry, DNA, RNA, hormones. The mind has been reduced in importance again. Yes, again. The massive interest in psychology that dominated (and still does in some respects) popular medicine since the 1950s arose as a reaction to the almost complete lack of interest in the mind shown by medicine in the preceding hundred years. The swing now to biochemistry is probably a reaction to the initial obsession with the mind.

Having said that, though, there still remains tremendous ignorance of the proper meaning of the term *psychosomatic* and its relationship to medicine, to psychology and to the newer theories of biochemistry. Saying something is psychosomatic *does not* mean that a physical event is *caused* by the mind. How I understand the term and will use it here, is that if an event in the physical – or somatic – realm involves *more* than the simplest of basic bodily activities, then the chances of higher bodily functions, especially brain or central nervous system functions being involved is very high. If this is the case, then it is probably true to say that we are then dealing with psychological functions as well. I equate higher brain functions with psychology. The terms themselves are, I believe, interchangeable but the levels of explanations of each discipline differs as do the methods of studying them.

Using this explanation then, it becomes clear that to say that something is psychosomatic is a convenient way of saying that a physical experience has higher-order brain or psychological causes that we think determine the experience. Headache is a physical pain felt in the head. The immediate *descriptive* cause of it is pain caused by muscle tension or blood flow disturbance but the *explanatory* cause is probably psychosomatic. This means simply that until we know the precise sequence of causes, we have to regard it as falling somewhere in the higher-brain and psychological functioning of the individual. After placing the area of most likely explanation, we have to attack the problem by coming at it from all sides – to see which psychological, physical, social and biochemical events cause, or get together to cause, headache. We must also be quite aware of how complex the problem is. If we find, for example, that histamine (a biochemical) causes headache (which it does) we have to avoid saying 'Aha, headaches are caused by histamine.' We have to ask instead: 'Now, what causes histamine to cause headache?' Likewise, if we find that migraine sufferers tend to be neat, obsessive perfectionists (which they seem to be) we have to avoid saying 'Perfectionism (a personality trait) causes headache.' Instead, we have to trace the specific links all the way from the perfectionist's upbringing down to the action of the blood vessels in his or her brain. Only then could we be sure that *all* non-organic headaches in *all* people are caused by perfectionism. What follows represents a statement about our current understanding of headache as a psychosomatic problem.

When you get a headache, several things happen all at or about the same time. The order of chain reaction seems to be as follows: Your physical or social environment upsets or disturbs

62

you. You react by activating your body in ways that we are as yet not clear about but, among other things, you activate your *autonomic* nervous system which transmits orders to your muscle and blood vessel networks. Prolonged and over-action of the former and disturbances in the latter cause pain to be registered back up in the higher nervous system (the *thalamus*). The role in this chain of the first two parts can easily be established because the same disturbances in blood vessels and muscle tensions – as, for example, when you play a sport or have a hot bath – do not necessarily cause pain to be registered. Now, either pain *is* registered when you play a game and your central nervous system ignores it (which it can choose to do) because its interests are directed elsewhere, or the nervous system has its own way of automatically coping at a low level with the stresses and changes involved. Depending on how severe the pain, both probably occur. A torn muscle is painful but people can override the pain. Normal stresses of exertion may reach high levels of pain but can be shut off if they get too great by spontaneous relaxation ordered by the central nervous system. What happens, then, in headache sufferers? Why does this not occur? More to the point – why does it occur in some people but not others and why at some times but not at others?

The answer is partially in the learning pattern that each person undergoes as he or she grows up. The pattern of automatically regulating the body while playing sport is not something the body does naturally. The child is born with the ability to do it, but it has to learn how to use that ability and most of us manage to do so. It is what we can call a 'safe-living cycle'. The bodily actions of the two components of the *autonomic* nervous system learn to work together in a safe, highly organised psychological, physical and social framework. The body learns to get aroused (using the *sympathetic* nervous system) and to relax (using the *para-sympathetic* nervous system), in certain clear and psycho-socially approved sequences, according to the hurly-burly of the game. Thus, getting excited, running, yelling, throwing, catching, even getting angry, crying or weeping are all co-ordinated both physically

63

and socially. In the space of any five minutes of any game, the body and the emotions go through a clear and complex sequence of events during which every individual arousal activity is paired with every other and likewise for the relaxing chain of events. Now imagine what would happen if elements of either of these chains were missing or were not permitted to occur for some reason or other. Imagine having to play a fast and furious game of football or ice-hockey *without* making a single sound. It gives me a headache just to think about it. The strain of restraining your mouth and jaw muscles – inhuman! And this is just, we think, what may happen to people who suffer from headache. Somewhere along the line between birth and adulthood, the normal sequence of emotional learning is interfered with either by a psychological disturbance in the psychological upbringing of the child or by some physical defect or trauma, both of which we infer can interfere with proper nervous system co-ordination.

The analogy of the football game or ice-hockey game is a useful one. It is an example of safe, institutionalised learning in which the growing child discovers how, to put it crudely, to put his or her body and mind together. There are many other situations which are very much less safe and less clear-cut and it is in these contexts that psychological problems can interfere with normal central nervous system co-ordinated learning. One example is the soundless football game described above. Sure, it's funny and hard to imagine but situations structurally just like this do occur very often in our daily lives. Your boss is rude to you and you are too scared to reply; someone criticises you and you clam up. You get infuriated by a newspaper report and rage inside, powerless to change things . . . It is very likely that these kinds of situations cause most of the headaches we collectively suffer. That is, these are the likely situations that cause our normal *autonomic* reactions to be interfered with.

So far so good. But what does it mean? Does this mean that we should go around shouting at each other, assaulting bosses or newspaper editors? Not quite. For a start, consider what

64

actually is stopping the normal chain of events, the normal physical sequence. Nothing in your own bodily make up, certainly. If I told you to play football soundlessly and you obeyed me, you'd be a fool, wouldn't you? But some people are brought up to have such a fear of authority, of public opinion, of appearing to cause trouble, that they will obey a command even if it means behaving in what is, for the nervous system, an abnormal way.

Having got this clear, let us now have a look at what the experts have had to say about what kinds of social and psychological contexts lead to such pathological learning occurring in headache-prone people.

Uncomplicated psychosomatic theories

One of the easy ways out of this explanatory dilemma is to put all your theoretical eggs in one basket. Headache is caused by your physical constitution, that is, it happens to tall, thin people with finely-chiselled features. This is one example of such a basket still thought to be true in some quarters today. More destructive, I think, has been the theory that headache, because it occurs (or seemed to occur) more often in women than men, has everything to do with female hormonal glands. Removal of uterus and/or ovaries was once prescribed in severe cases, not with altogether satisfactory results.

Getting back to more strictly psychosomatic theories though, as was to be expected the psychotherapists have had a field day with headache and migraine. Headache has been related to birth trauma (you get headache according to the kind of birth you had), to early experiences of parental 'primality' (love-making) and to an unconscious identification with the genitalia in which the feelings of head swelling, splitting and so on are simply the acts of the person transferring the sensations of a forbidden part of the body to a more socially accept-able one – the head. The idea behind all of these is that exposure to certain traumatic incidents (birth, parental sex, one's own sexual desires) had so upset the person that any-thing that reminded him or her of the original trauma would

5

cause a headache. For one writer, the migraine patient's blocking of his or her visual field is due to an attempt to unconsciously shut off the offending image. So there you have it.

There have been less doctrinaire attempts to explain the psychology of headache. Clinic workers noted early that their headache and migraine patients suffered from a range of other psychological problems that seemed to help to analyse their cause. Headache people are highly ambitious, for example, rigid and controlled in their behaviour and, of course, perfectionists. Along with this goes a poorly-developed ability to express emotions, especially anger and hostility. The clinical picture is of a conscientious person with drive who likes to be liked, to be approved of, works hard and meticulously at whatever goal he or she thinks would bring approval and, in the process, fails to express normal tension and anger for fear of disapproval. Headache is the inevitable result.

People with highly developed histories of headache such as chronic headache and migraine sufferers, seem to come from families in which prestige, pride and convention run hand in glove with subservience and authoritarianism. This ensures that the growing child both obeys the family ethic and feels in some way he or she can't cope. Anger and frustration at this failure, together with fear of exposing the failure, causes the headache symptom. Some experts regard this symptom as a means of self-punishment for daring to be angry and frustrated in the first place. Others regard it as an inability to tolerate stress and frustration – the anger and hostility arising because the person feels hurt and petulant at the lack of instant approval or gratification for his or her needs.

All very interesting, but go through the descriptions carefully and you will find that most people would probably fit quite well into the patterns. Most of us are ambitious, like to please people, love attention and approval and try not to make too much fuss in general. Very few people go around openly expressing hostility and anger and most of us have some trouble expressing negative emotions like anger anyway. What makes chronic headache sufferers different from those who don't have many headaches or who are headache-free? And how do we explain ambitious, compulsive, driving, upright types who never get a headache? Why headaches at some times and not others? These are just general questions that have to be answered before more detailed inquiries are made, such as how does the failure to express anger actually, physically or biochemically, cause headache?

Research on trying to establish a headache or migraine type of personality has as yet not even got to the first general set of questions. While most studies have found that migraine and chronic headache subjects do tend to be more disturbed (more neurotic, more obsessional, but not, it seems, more anxious) quite how and why this is related to both personality and the physiology of head pain is not clear. It is widely presumed, for example, that the pain itself – the muscular tension and blood vessel disturbance – occurs as the person struggles to control or, rather, repress his or her hostility. Research has not, however, been able to establish that chronic sufferers have more re-pressed hostility than either occasional sufferers or non-sufferers. Given the physical differences between muscle-contraction and migraine headache, one would presume that personality or psychological factors associated with each would also differ. Yet the only reliably known difference is that tension headache sufferers tend to show more anxiety than migraine sufferers (Gainotti et al, 1972).

There is another problem which these uncomplicated theories tend to overlook: most of the research has been done on *patients* – people who have got so desperate they have sought help from a clinic or a psychotherapist. People who suffer from any kind of pain for a long time tend to get obsessional, depressed, resentful, angry, frustrated – the lot. It is quite possible that these traits not only may arise as a *result* of having headache but that they may in fact have nothing to do with the *cause* of headache. While some of the data obtained from studies of extreme sufferers is obviously of value, it must be remembered that they obscure the fact that we know very little indeed about ordinary headache and ordinary migraine.

As we saw earlier in the book, when a really good study comes along – like Water's Pontypridd survey – a whole lot of firmly-held convictions (like the relationship between social class and intelligence) are found to have no grounding in reality. Bearing this in mind, let us now have a look at what a complex psychosomatic theory might look like.

Towards a complex psychosomatic theory

For a start, it is probably best not to think in terms of a headache or migraine type of personality nor to try to relate concepts like anger or hostility, perfectionism or obsessionality to things which cause headache. They are all too gross, too large, too unwieldy. Not even researchers who have specialised in specific areas like anger are agreed upon a precise meaning for the terms they use. It is far better, I think, to stick fairly close to what is both reliably known and can be adequately explained. Put simply, it is no good saying, for example, 'Headaches are caused by repressed hostility'. You have to supply the chain of possible or hypothetical actions which link the two. So, going back to the chain of contributory events we began this chapter with, let's start at the top and work down to the chemistry of the nerves.

Society. Most sane adults would agree that human societies have problems. By far the most important concerns the question of how relationships between each individual and each social group should be conducted. Since time began, men and women have been alternately beating the hell out of one another and making friends. In its specific geographical, political and social context each different society and each different era has created its own rules for conducting the twin activities of fighting and living in peace. So when we are born, we arrive into a context that to some extent is already set for us. Of course, we may be a budding Adolf Hitler and have our own view of conflicts but, by and large, we learn the broad rules laid down by our society. Thus Australians express their anger by throwing beer cans, Greeks tend to sing revolutionary songs very angrily, Germans get haughty and polite and Britons? . . . well, somewhere between writing letters to the newspapers and tearing up goal posts. There is no truth, incidentally, in the rumour that the incidence of headache in Britain increased during the absence of *The Times*, nor that building more protective fences in football grounds has meant more headache for soccer fans.

Now, the reason that war and peace arise is that the ideal requirements for human bodily function are not readily available on the earth as it has been so far organised. At the simplest level, each organism needs an adequate supply of material (psychological and physical) to fill such basic needs as eating and drinking. Each individual, therefore, learns a set of priorities about how and what needs are to be filled according to the position his family occupies in the general rush to get at the available resources.

What concerns us here is *how* we learn those social rules because certain societies and eras have generated rules that do not accord very well with the basic psychological and nerve requirements of the human organism. Even if a society or an era has a healthy set of rules, it is possible for individuals – often large numbers of individuals – to learn the rules in a faulty way. What, then, constitutes faulty learning? And what do we mean by 'faulty learning'? Faulty rules are, of course, of interest in precipitating certain conditions (we could argue, for instance, that the pace of modern life sets up the conditions for headache) but they aren't the real issue because individuals do not *have* to accept the rules of their society. What matters is under what *conditions* do people *choose* to ignore the signs of their own bodies that health problems are occurring? And herein lies a possible answer to the question of what constitutes faulty learning. As a general but rough rule, anything that causes human discomfort in the act of living is 'bad' for the organism, whether or not the fault lies in the social rules he or she learns or mislearns. Thus, although we live in a highly pressured and intensely competitive world, the real issue is *why* do we conform to it *if* part of the result of such conformity is discomfort such as headache? What, in other words, interferes with the normal body tendency to minimise discomfort and pain?

Families. The answer to this might well lie in how families bring up their children. We learn our rules, how to deal with cohabitation and conflict in our families and it is here that problems of interpretation might occur. It is here that we may be *forced* to conform to a rule that doesn't make sense – like having to play a football game in silence. Again the problem is not in the rule itself, but how we learn it. Most of us are able (or free enough) to recognise bad rules when we see them or to recognise bad ways of being taught. What we do about it is crucial – how we cope, in other words, with recognising that something is wrong and *not* allowing ourselves to suffer in the process, determines our level of adjustment – our own individual way of conflict and living together.

Individuals. Basically, it all comes down to *you*, the individual. If there is no organic base for such physical discomforts as headache then, logically, you choose to tolerate head pain when physically you shouldn't. Why should this be? The newborn child arrives in a state of relative unsophistication. Not only does the infant have an undeveloped nervous system, but it also has a high degree of flexibility. It is open to literally hundreds of possible avenues to develop along and, more importantly, to learning many different types of organisation. It is quite easy for a baby to learn a whole set of nervous interconnections without ever realising that they may be abnormal. In particular, he or she may learn a level of pain or frustration that, in terms of our rough model of physical discomfort, is intolerable. This is terribly important. The act of healthy survival means you must manage cohabitation and conflict comfortably. By that, I don't mean lazily, I mean by sensible and selective choices. If you decide to tolerate pain, for example, it is for a *set* time or *set* purpose – not as a way of life. To do this the individual must be able not only to hear (or feel) his sensory input tell him or her that something is wrong, but also to act on the warning signs sensibly. We all have this function and when it is disturbed, it means that the individual or child has learned to systematically ignore a certain level of pain. More particularly, it has learnt to organise its system in such a way that a whole set of alarm-raising body functions are ignored because his or her social environment does not permit the child to react to them properly.

Central nervous system organisation.
To get a headache involves quite a sophisticated series of activities in the central nervous system. A lot of *autonomic* lower-order 'healthy' – or stabilising – operations have to be overridden. The body has to be, as it were, thrown into reverse by our idiot of a driver. If we think of a growing child we can see this clearly. The central or higher nervous system organisation is loose and unsophisticated, but the lower activities of the nervous system are quite well established and efficient. These allow the child's basic activities to function without thought or environmental interference, apart from succour and warmth. Thus while the child can't organise its perceptions or think in an organised way, his or her heart beats well, blood flows comfortably, defecation, urination, eating and sleeping all take place normally. To get headache – which very young children do *not* seem to get – demands that some of these regulatory activities be inverted and subordinated to the new requirements made by the environment on the central nervous system. The child actually *learns* to introduce pain into his or her life when previously it was absent.

If we stop there, it is clear that already we have woven a fascinating web of intriguing questions without drawing on simple ideas of explanation and without ignoring the need to integrate the many levels that contribute to the development of headache. More important for what follows, we have established a multi-levelled way of looking at headache that allows you, the individual, to contribute to your own inquiry about your headache, its causes, origin and its possible cure. Let me explain how.

This overall framework says three essential things about the

71

cause of headache. First, it says that you have imposed your headache organisation on your ordinary level of central nervous system activity. Technically, if you imposed it, you can remove it. Secondly, it says that you may (and I believe it is highly possible) be unaware of how you did it and why, because it was ingrained or, more correctly, integrated with your psychological functioning at an early age. Thirdly, it says that the clues as to how and why will lie in several possible areas concurrently – in your social surroundings, in your family, in your individual personality and in the functioning of your central nervous system. Any one of these levels can be used by you to explore the headache and to modify or improve it. Depending on your determination and your desire to get better, it is possible to use these keys to introduce your body to a wide range of possibilities which, if applied sensibly and thoughtfully, could by-pass the need to find an actual cause.

If you get headaches, you will naturally want to get rid of them. What I intend doing in the rest of this book, therefore, is to examine and explore the various treatment options using this complex model in order that *you* can see what can be done at each level – social, family, individual, neural and bio-chemical. You will also see what each level implies and what the treatments imply – ie, what they can and cannot do, what side-effects and dangers attend them and so on – and where you can contribute to organise your treatment and your understanding better. You, in other words, are going to be put slap-bang in the middle of the picture so that you can get on with the job of researching and fixing your own headache.

CHAPTER EIGHT

Migraine people

Some people get constructive headache that they put up with to achieve certain results. Applying for a raise or deciding to have an argument with the grocer may cause you a headache. If you carry out your decision and/or achieve your goal, it is well worth the pain. In this respect, headache is perfectly normal and acceptable. When, however, you aren't *directing* your headache, when the head pain just happens or when the balance between normal and abnormal occurrences becomes disproportionately high, then your headache has become an integral part of your day-to-day life. The most extreme example of this is migraine. We can start our examination by looking at how our model of psychosomatic functioning applies to migraine people, because if we can understand migraine, we will be in a better position to understand less well-organised headache. Because of its severity, more is known about migraine and nearly all the treatment methods, especially the drugs used, have been developed for migraine rather than for headache.

If a simple headache acts for the body as a warning that something is wrong, then migraine is what the body does if the mind or higher brain centres ignore the warning. Put simply, migraine is a highly efficient fail-safe system whereby the body takes the necessary action to stop whatever you were doing and take evasive action. In a strange and apparently unorthodox manner, it is possible to regard migraine not solely as a crippling illness, but as a highly organised safety mechanism.

This somewhat inverted view of migraine is one that

emerges both from clinical experience and from what has been reliably established by research. It is also one that allows the complex levels of analysis we raised in Chapter 7 to be applied with some degree of comfort. To do this, I want to consider each level separately, inverting the order and starting with the central nervous system and its organisation in the child and then examining what happens in the individual, the family and society.

Childhood origins of migraine

Most physicians and pediatricians would probably agree that outside the usual childhood illnesses, children have little access to channels of communication for acknowledging puzzling or confusing internal states. For one thing they lack the knowledge of their right to both relief from distress and to express it; and for another, they lack adequate language. This is especially the case when the child has to transfer from a highly efficient way of expressing discomfort – crying and yelling – to the far more sophisticated but not so natural act of talking. To scream or yell or cry when we are distressed is a primitive response in which the gap between discomfort and expression is slight and neatly co-ordinated by the twin routes of the central nervous system – the *sympathetic* and *para-sympathetic* systems. Talking involves much higher nervous system activity and it is very likely that the introduction of this demand by the child's parents creates the kind of stress and interference in central nervous system activity that we spoke about in the last chapter.

In a normal child, this transitory phase is usually introduced over quite a long time so that the 'baby' responses of crying and yelling are slowly integrated with the new verbal responses. At the same time the child is able to develop his or her own intermediary steps, like half-crying and half-yelling, partly reassuring him or herself, knowing when to run to mummy, when to brave it out and when to cry.

What happens if the transition is faulty, if the child is *expected* to talk instead of act, 'You're five now, start talking and stop crying'? Obviously a whole possible range of stresses can arise. The child might struggle to conform, might break down, might develop other symptoms such as bed-wetting (more about these symptoms a little later). Migraine children appear to fit into this pattern in that their preliminary symptoms show them to be confused and mixed up as if their world has been turned upside-down and they don't know why; as if they are being expected to be or do something that is beyond them. They show more clearly than any type of adult sufferer of either headache or migraine that a disintegration of nervous system functioning occurs *before* the actual onset of head pain. Clinical reports indicate that such children start off with an acute *confusional* disturbance in which they are unable to answer their parents' questions or commands, get apprehensive, agitated, disorientated and show a strange form of anger. They seem ready to strike out at anything (Ehyai and Fenichel, 1978).

Other research has established that nausea or related stomach and intestinal disturbances almost always accompany headache in children who later develop migraine (Bo Bille, 1968). Car or travel (really, motion) sickness is also a frequent preceding symptom in childhood. More important, it is clear that the children involved in the studies did not tell their parents in detail about their disturbances. The investigator was often the first to discover the nature and extent of the problem.

These findings suggest that the children studied were both frightened and, in an important respect, neglected by their parents. When they are frightened, children tend to cry or run to their parents for physical reassurance. When these outlets are not permitted, the next most common form of expressing fear is by the use of stomach and intestinal symptoms such as runny tummy, nausea, vomiting and so on. The migraine child is *not* emotionally or materially neglected by the parents – far from it. They are often a central part of the family life and great attention is often focused on the child. The child's coping responses are, however, ignored. In migraine boys, for example, I have found that parents inevitably have missed the child's earlier signs of confusion and upset because they were ashamed or embarrassed by them and were even too afraid to tell their family doctor. In many cases I was able to discover only after months of investigation that parents often found their little sons had frequently become unaccountably upset when watching television or movies. We will see the significance of this in a moment.

What adds weight to the argument that this combination of fear and neglect may contribute to the disintegration of central nervous system functioning is the fact that migraine children I have studied earlier on in their lives developed quite normal crying and yelling. It was in fact the parents who had changed their demands when they felt the child should have outgrown his or her 'baby' behaviour. I have also found parents of migraine children to be much harder emotionally on their children than non-migraine but headache-prone children. They are also more unaccepting of stress symptoms in themselves.

To complete the picture, a recent study at the St Louis Children's Hospital in the United States (Prensky and Sommer, 1979) found a whole range of other accompanying stress symptoms in the children studied. Some were over-active, others couldn't pay attention for long, were compulsive, anxious and had problems at school. Many were depressed and not as a result of getting headache. Bo Bille's study, cited earlier, reported incidentally that children with migraine were absent from school more often than other children (and not for reasons of migraine). Perfectionistic, hard, driving, ambitious children or children under an enormous degree of stress? I think stress has it; and the most likely cause seems to be that these children are struggling to express discomfort and 'emotional pain' through language but because it is an adult language and has no room for 'childishness', it doesn't do the job. At the same time they cannot take a step backwards to more childish forms of behaviour.

It is this latter point that I think may complete the chain in childhood central nervous system collapse and help us explain why headache as a way of expressing distress takes place in some children under stress but not others. When growing children hit problems and they can't talk about them properly, they usually regress. They become babies again or childish or infantile; they bed-wet, cling, have nightmares, suck their thumbs and so on. They are scared or frightened and to cope they resort to an old but acceptable way of behaving. Headache and migraine children don't do this – they don't appear to allow themselves the 'luxury' of regression.

Regression is a natural way the body has of managing stress. Psychologically and physically, as stress mounts, the body naturally falls back on to modes of behaviour that previously acted either to remove the stress or to protect the child from it. If the first old pattern tried does not produce the required results, the body systematically regresses to progressively lower levels of functioning until one works. What seems to happen in migraine children is that none of the 'normal' regressive patterns work. The most severe signs of distress are eventually resorted to, hence all the symptoms of central nervous system disintegration we have described above. As you can see, headache and migraine in children are really the child's final fail-safe system at work – they at last ensure that the environment provides the necessary attention. A child can't help itself properly (even though some children do try) so it signals to its environment to do so.

Next, we have to relate this form of activity to the kind of basic neural (nerve-system) processes that may be at work in the migraine child. Let us assume we are dealing with an emotionally fragile child, which the research evidence suggests we are, and one who is easily physically upset by change – either in the sense of simple motion change, as in travelling, or more social changes, like going to school and learning new skills. It is very likely that such a child functions in a highly specific stereotyped way; in other words he or she responds to stress in the same way each time. For one thing, his or her general level of arousal would probably be unstable, that is, have no stable basic pattern, having recently had to change from a deeply satisfying one to a far less stable one. Second, since one of the

77

overriding functions of any biological system is to achieve a stable state of relatively constant input and output, it is quite likely that the child would seize on anything constant. Thus you would get a child who, in shifting from a 'baby' way of expressing stress to an adult, spoken one, would focus, perhaps obsessively, on superficial signs that apparently ease stress. A child struggling with the shift would, for example, be disproportionately pleased by a good word or grade at school and be excessively distressed by a bad word or failure. No child or nervous system can go on for so long at this high level of fear or anxiety. No sensitive system can cope with the constant stress of looking and watching for the slightest signs of encouragement or disapproval. Such a child would have a nervous system that would function like a loaded gun, waiting for just one more thing – one more upset – to go off.

It is very important to realise the significant role played by the environment in the development of a child's nervous system. As we have said, the child's brain at birth is highly flexible and the key to understanding the shape of growth lies in the pattern of organisation it adopts to cope with its own needs and those of the environment. Precisely the same is true of the patterns that make up migraine. A child learns to co-ordinate and organise what are initially random and unrelated movements, nerve impulses, responses, thoughts and feelings (as in playing a game) through environmental and self-induced feedback (*'Watch* the ball, you idiot!). In precisely the same way, the same structure is employed to put together the various components that together make up a proneness to migraine.

The scene thus set, let us see what happens as the child grows older.

Individuality and adolescence in the development of migraine
The effect of actually having a migraine attack is considerable and not just on the child. In a strange and tragic way, it serves to organise and explain a set of phenomena that have often, for months, disturbed and distressed the child, his parents, doctors and teachers. At last, all is clear – 'You have migraine, dear,' a

78

mother or father will say, 'that's all. And that's why you've been so upset and doing so badly at school.' And of course, the doctor and school teacher will doubtless confirm the parents' attitude and all will breathe a sigh of relief. All happily and blithely confusing the effect with the cause. Migraine does not cause distress – distress causes migraine. This is a crucial but often ignored distinction. Of course, migraine *is* unpleasant but what causes it in the first place is doubly distressing and it is this that must be put back in our thinking about migraine.

Take the child who has an attack. It always follows after a fairly long period of anguish made desperate by the lack of adequate recognition. In itself, it is a terrifying experience. Having had the puzzle explained as 'migraine' and wishing to avoid both the preceding period and a recurrence of the attack, the child attempts to relate it to something that happened at or about the same time. This is a natural enough tendency helped along by parents and other 'authorities' who point at simple occurrences instead of looking at the complexity involved. So the child pays attention to whatever seemed to trigger the attack and this is usually something like bright lights, *watching television*, a test at school and the like – all reasons cited in Bo Bille's study. It can, of course, be food or smoke or something similar.

Because watching out for such simple things is easy for both parent and child, hey presto! a very strange thing happens. The child suddenly begins to get attention he or she didn't get before, or the parents actually begin to *help* avoid the things thought to bring on migraine – 'Don't sit too close to the set, dear – don't want you to get migraine again.' So, at last, the child has found a regressive system that works. In my opinion, whether or not a migraine pattern becomes entrenched depends on how effectively constructed this new framework is. In some families, the first migraine attack so shakes the parents up that they genuinely attend to the child and, in so doing, remove the complex determining conditions. In families with histories of migraine, though, the parents tend to toss the whole thing off – 'It's just migraine, we know all about it'. And this is why, I think, children born into migraine families tend to have migraine. An attack is neither unexpected nor disturbing and gets no special attention, so they continue.

In other individuals, the attacks may lift quite spontaneously due to fluctuations in parental moods, teacher support and so on, only to reappear at a later stage when a new and disrupting set of conditions arise – notably with the trauma of adolescence. Either way, what remains is a vulnerable and unstable personality and central nervous system which must now concern us.

What happens to a child who develops migraine as a child or adolescent and it becomes an established part of his or her life? To understand this, we have to first distinguish between the underlying physical conditions that we described earlier *and* the added conditions created by the act of *having* migraine. This distinction is often omitted in treatises on migraine, and I believe this has helped to create so much confusion about the condition because what individuals *often* do with their migraine attacks, especially in their adolescence and adulthood, is to use them as a means of expressing passive hostility and anger. Then, like any patient with a disability, the disability becomes a tool with its own history and movement quite apart from the underlying *actual* physical condition and its causes. Complexes built on complexes, if you like.

What recurrent migraine attacks do to the basic central nervous system in the child is essentially to freeze its level of functioning at onset of migraine. Once the pattern of attacks is established, there is very little that the child can do to either unfreeze his or her functioning or to improve and restabilise the mechanisms at a more efficient level. I have frequently found with patients recovering from migraine attacks – that is, when therapy has broken their patterns – that they are left with a level of functioning that is best described as child-like or adolescent-like, depending on when the pattern was first established. I have known forty or fifty-year-old people have almost child-like obsessions and preoccupations (such as I described earlier) of almost unbelievable proportions. This, too, might

80

well account for the list of attributes migraine people are supposed to have – such as a simple perfectionism, a child-like rigidity and so on. They are all ways of personal and neural functioning more commonly found in children and adolescents.

Why this freezing process occurs is fairly easily seen. To get migraine in the first place means that the child lives in a deprived environment. The only way he or she is going to *really* get better is if the parents and child are taught or shown how to correct the child's disturbances properly – that is, through their interaction and their sensitivity to what actually causes it. Since I know of no social treatment or advice programme that focuses on this, I presume that in chronic cases it does not occur. The child *cannot* change unless his or her environment changes its pattern of sensing and reacting to needs. Hence the big freeze.

What happens after this is interesting and depends to a certain extent on how the child and family react to the attacks and what influences in the environment operate on the child. In chronic migraine people, the *aftermath* of migraine lays a level of functioning on top of the original disorder and you get the familiar patterns we associate with migraine developing. Sufferers become concerned with avoiding attacks, with avoiding stimuli that they think cause an attack, with finding new or better drugs, with trying different treatment methods and so on. They form relationships inside and outside the family that are based on migraine and its condition – relationships which either reduce their migraine or which guarantee them a continuation of whatever happened at home. It all depends on how extensive attacks are, how they are treated and what opportunities exist in the person's environment to modify the basic, underlying condition.

So let's forget for a moment about the kind of 'sufferer' pattern or syndrome and concentrate on what it means to have a frozen personal and neural structure.* At the basic level, it

* Migraine produces secondary gain through the sufferer demanding sympathy and expecting to be excused from arduous tasks or treated as a 'special case'; given privileges and protection not really relevant to the

means that the growing child has established a very restrictive and inflexible personal and physical system which continues to direct his or her activity in every aspect of their lives. The child's personality is not organised around avoiding migraine. In both childhood and adolescence migraine is a fairly isolated stress reaction which alternates with long headache-free periods. The basic malfunction (difficulty in coping with stress) and the family tensions that result under extreme circumstances in migraine, become the base round which the child's personality is organised. Thus all new experience to the individual with this frozen system is analysed and organised in terms of the malfunction. Experiences do not allow the child to grow much or to change and do not act – as they should – as shapers of the individual. Bear in mind, I am talking about chronic sufferers. Each individual will have some areas of their own functioning that do adapt and change and give individual differences. What is central, though, is that in coping with stress, much the same patterns will be common to all migraine sufferers because of the frozen development in that area.

Now, where is this deficit likely to show? Each individual will have his or her own specific areas learnt in the family. They will tend to be characterised by a concern with appearance instead of reality, an inability to see depth and relativity and anxiety that is not based on specific content. This means that what causes stress may differ from person to person but it will always arise because of an inability of the person to see reality properly. They will always relate reality to their frozen structure and if insurmountable and unavoidable conflict arises, migraine will result. It is these twin tendencies that will determine when and where migraine develops. Thus, any situation the person finds both inescapable and stressful will create migraine. Hence exam stresses, school work stresses, inescapable social stresses such as watching movies and attending

basic problem involved. It is these secondary gains that lead to problems such as passive hostility, latent anger and so on. While important, I don't think they are as important as the primary level of migraine problem which we will concentrate on.

dinner parties and, above all, stresses in relationships, particularly to close relations. The growing child will thus suffer periods of relief and stress according to the ebb and flow of such experiences. The child whose migraine disappears when he moves school or passes an exam may not have changed his basic make up but simply have moved out of the orbit of stress for a time. In the same way, a person leaving home may stop migraine attacks induced by parental stress but find them reoccurring later in a marriage in which the stress is duplicated.

Family and social contributions to migraine pathology
Right at the start of this part of the discussion, we talked about the twin 'basic' problems of organising conflict and living together. These are all-embracing structures that can be said to describe the human condition. It is in the family and later in society that these basic problems arise. What you learn in your family, so you apply and modify and maybe re-learn outside in society. Social contexts are therefore *human* contexts, which throw up problems of conflict and agreement. Life is, if you like, a series of battles which you can win or lose. What concerns us here is what happens to the migraine structure as it meets these problems.

To answer this, let's outline broadly what these battles are. First, the growing child has to separate from its parents and live on its own. Second, it has to form friendships of its own. Third, it has to form an intimate relationship with a member of the opposite sex. And fourth, it has to bear children and raise its own family. Along the way, of course, it has also to develop its own ability to work, hold a job and so on. This is the fifth battle. Probe a migraine person's adjustment closely and you should, if our basic model is correct, find problems in each of these five areas, organised around the frozen personal and neural development. That is, we should find that the migraine person tends to approach each superficially and when put under stress, develops migraine. Not all areas will operate at the same time and problems or exposure in any one can cause migraine. This is why it is a mistake to look for specific

83

situations that cause migraine. You have to consider the whole complex web of causes as we have done in this chapter.

The evidence both from clinical and research studies in my opinion demonstrates very clearly that this is precisely what happens to migraine people. They tend to have the following:

(a) They are over-involved with their parents and original home ties long after they should have broken emotionally from home. Parents, or other close family members continue to have considerable undue influence and effect. A visit to any one – mother, father, sister or brother – provokes stress or conflict.

(b) They tend to form unsatisfactory relationships, having superficial acquaintances rather than deep friendships. These friendships are characterised by clear stages. An initial one in which the migraine person is terribly enthusiastic about the 'new' friend, and a later one in which hurt, frustration, disappointment and anger (always expressed to someone else – not the friend involved) predominate. The person always returns to the bosom of the family after these ventures outside.

(c) The marital partner chosen or, rather, the person that the migraine sufferer seems to end up with is nearly always of a certain kind – someone who is prepared to accept or live with a very reduced sense of intimacy. My studies on this phenomenon are as yet incomplete but what is clear so far is that the non-migraine partner in such a relationship nearly always has personal deficiencies not related to headache. This finding applies more where the relationship has been long lasting, usually over five years. The non-migraine partner seems patient, kind, understanding, shy even. But underneath this they are usually extracting enormous benefits from the relationship by concealing their own inadequacy, underdevelopment and fear. I have yet to find a chronic migraine sufferer who has a healthy relationship with his or her partner. The two, I think, are incompatible.

(d) Having children and all it involves in chronic migraine sufferers is, on close examination, a traumatic experience full of 'special case' problems. It is not so much the actual act of having children or the material looking after them but the anxiety attached to them and their future. The children are overprotected and are worried about in the wrong way. They are cosseted, admonished, treated like little dolls, as precious objects to be kept neat, clean and tidy.

(e) The migraine person's ability to hold a job or to be competent is not to be faulted; what is, though, is his or her level of intellectual functioning. They appear to be quick-witted, intelligent, alert and conscientious but this is purely a *socially* learned set of activities. Very few chronic migraine patients show real creative intelligence, originality or a sustained ability to direct their own thinking. They tend to have learned how to give the impression of intelligence, to be conscientious and so on. In reality, they soon tire if praise and encouragement is not constantly forthcoming. In my opinion, they often may have real talent or intelligence but will only use it if pushed and 'mothered' all the way.

The point of all this is that, where families and societies contribute to the migraine pattern, it is very easy for the migraine person to survive without realising something is wrong. We tolerate and accept migraine as a piece of bad luck, as something that has nothing to do with the individual or his family. And this is where we go wrong. The contribution of parents in a migraine person's family has already been discussed. What remains is to pin-point where societies go wrong.

It should be easy, as we said earlier, to blame society for such things as stress, rush, urban chaos, competitiveness and so on, but this really does miss the point. What we, as a society, have neglected – certainly in this century – is a correct appreciation of how to manage the twin problems of cohabitation and conflict. Think how a growing child or adolescent learns how to argue or fight properly, how to debate or discuss coherently, how and when to compromise, how to be tolerant. All he or she has to go on is scraps of information picked up from odd books, newspaper or magazine articles, visuals from films or television (never the best place to observe reality) and perhaps glimpses of mum and dad having a fight. The rest is gained from friends and their own personal experience which is often a case of the blind leading the blind. So long as things seem all right on the surface, how is any individual to know that something fundamental is wrong? If a family goes wrong as in migraine, if doctors and society don't recognise the depth of the problem, there is no way of correcting the public's misconceptions. The art of living has been neglected and many millions of people are expected to survive in the most serious and intimate of relationships with very little proper basic information about either the problems involved or what is required from them. We spend more time teaching children about birth control than we do about how to bring up children properly or how to relate to one another. Little wonder that today people are desperate for information and constantly seek advice about how to live and how to relate. It is this kind of lack of knowledge that is society's contribution to migraine.

Last word on migraine

Having said all that about migraine, I now have to say that this represents the extreme pole of the headache syndrome. The range of headaches that occur in between this and the simple, constructive headache described at the beginning of the chapter contain varying degrees of this extreme structure. So it is quite possible that what has been said here only applies to part of the functioning of other people who have headache. Muscle contraction or tension headache, for example, is a far less well-organised phenomenon, but it does have many of the components of the migraine organisation and it certainly serves a similar, if less extreme, function. In time we will, I feel sure, tease out the precise pattern of these headaches. But as yet, this is not possible.

The central point is that if headache becomes chronic, whatever its form, then it can be said with a high degree of certainty that the sufferer's central nervous system, his or her personality *and* their personal relationships, are all involved in the process and all contain a degree of the symptoms we have sketched in this chapter. While the amount of physical suffering involved is not to be ignored, the extent of emotional suffering is far more extensive and widespread than is generally appreciated. Let us now, therefore, turn in the remainder of the book, to see what can be done about both these aspects of headache and migraine.

CHAPTER NINE

Treatment 1: Muscle-contraction (tension) headache

With such a complex and multi-faceted problem as headache, there are obviously many ways of approaching treatment. What we will do in this chapter, is examine these ways and then, in Chapters 11, 12 and 13, look at the possibility of *cure* as opposed to simply treatment.

As things stand now, we have inherited a range of treatment options based more on the economics of the chemical industry than the demands of the conditions involved. I say this because there are two really highly efficient treatment methods known to man which have no side-effects, always work and can be used time and time again without losing their effectiveness. Neither involves chemicals and neither has been attended to much, either by researchers or victims. Not surprising. The first is sleep – the most efficient and the cheapest method, but hardly marketable. The second is the gravitational accelerator used to accustom astronauts to the high forces of gravity they experience on lift-off. Got a headache? Then do a James Bond and risk a twirl in an accelerator and sample the benefits of the world's most expensive but highly efficient cure for headache. We won't return to the accelerator but we will have a look at sleep later.

For non-astronauts there is a choice of a variety of drugs, many of which promise relief from headache and some which just claim to help ease the pain. What I want to do is to examine the available methods and try to give a realistic assessment of what they can and cannot do. The thing to remember about the methods used in the treatment of headache and migraine conditions is that they each constitute one line of attack on an essentially highly complex problem. Their effectiveness has to be evaluated in terms of whether they do the job they are supposed to do and what contribution they make to the problem as a whole. Then, the question has to be asked, 'How can the method be better used in the treatment of headache?' In other words, what can the patient (or his doctor) do to improve the effectiveness of both the method chosen to be used and the process of selecting that method. In what follows, we will focus on a *realistic* assessment of all these factors rather than presenting a simple list of the available methods. I will presume, incidentally, that having read the early chapters of the book, you know what kind of psychological and social headache you possess.

Treating tension or muscle-contraction headache
The first thing to do if you suffer from tension headache and can clearly differentiate it from migraine, is to decide how much of your physical and personal functioning is involved. Is it a temporary, one-off kind of experience or is it a more routine, more frequent occurrence? Can it be related to any specific event or do they just seem to creep up on you for no clear reason? The answers to these questions usually determine the choice of treatment. We will assume that occasional headache is neither here nor there and will concentrate on moderate frequency headache and chronic headache.

Moderate frequency tension headaches don't generally involve too much of the individual's neural or personal systems and may in fact be a simple warning device that it's time to ease the load on your body. How you can best do this depends on what you are doing at the time. Without question, the *best* thing to do is to sleep. Quite apart from the fact that all but the most chronic of headaches respond to sleep, many people cannot relax their bodies properly without sleeping. They have not learnt to develop self-control of phases of their conscious activity and so need big social signs to tell them to do so. They get up at the same time each day, eat at the same time and it is the same with sleep. You will be surprised how many people can only sleep at a designated time and for whom the idea of cat-napping at odd hours or sleeping during the day is impossible.

If you can't sleep, either because you have never got into the habit or because your job, spouse, children or whatever won't allow it, you can try several things. The most usual is to take one of the many analgesics on the market. Popular pain killers like aspirin seem to work for many people and if they work for you when you get occasional headache, well and good. What do you do, though, if pain killers either don't work or only partially work or, worse, they work but the side-effects cause you more trouble than the headache? Side-effects are quite a consideration for many people who just don't ordinarily like feeling drugged or nauseous and for others who can't perform as well if their equilibrium is just the slightest bit disturbed.

You can try shopping around for a better pain killer for your personal needs. Chats to your doctor or chemist may help guide you as to what precise products are available but they won't be able to help all that much because quite why some people prefer one drug to another is not clear. There are newer products than aspirin such as phenacetin, paracetamol, pentazocine and codeine (these are the common names – ask for them from your chemist and he will tell you what each's *trade* name is) and also many different types of combinations of the basic chemicals. Each drug you try should be investigated carefully by you and your doctor. Codeine, for example, can constipate you; aspirin can't be taken in some medical conditions or if you are on certain other forms of medication. It has also been linked to gastric irritation and, in some cases, gastric erosion. Other drugs have unpleasant side-effects or can be dangerous if only slightly misused, as for instance, if you overdose yourself. Paracetamol, phenacetin and codeine come into this category. Paracetamol has hepatotoxic effects; Phenacetin is being phased out in some countries and its use minimised in certain countries but *not* in others. (If in doubt remember that as a rough rule the American and British drug control councils take a tougher line than some others.) These drugs cause kidney damage and interfere with certain functions of the blood if misused.

Pain killers are the first line of attack generally recommended by your doctor. But there is another which may interest you – the use of various kinds of vitamins either taken orally or by injection. Some people have reported good results on this way of reducing headaches but so far there have been few studies that have tested their effectiveness in general. There are even some studies that show vitamin use up in a bad light, although not with headaches but with overdosing and taking non-naturally prepared vitamins. The best thing to do is see your doctor and ask his advice. Some people respond better than others and your doctor will be able to guide you.

You might incidentally like to try muscle-relaxant drugs. They may work but, in general, they are not reputed to be highly effective. Some people prefer taking effervescent tablets, so bear this in mind when you're experimenting. Personally, I have found that a great many psychological factors enter into the act of drug-taking and these can be as responsible as any other factor in the final preference. Some people can't stand even the vague taste of a tablet and for them, an injection of exactly the same chemicals has a very different effect.

Psychological factors also enter into what you do with the drug you are going to use. You may find a certain drug works and then swear by it for ever-after, yet a combination of psychological events could have ensured that you used the drug properly. For example, if you take a rest *after* taking a pain killer, you greatly improve the chances of it helping you. So, on one occasion you might try a new pill and just by chance take a rest as well. You attribute your pain relief to the new pill when it may be due to the pill plus rest, or rest alone, or your state of mind plus rest. The body is a great storer and collector of low-level information especially when it concerns its own well-being. When you come to use that pill again, the

91

idea of using it alone may well act to relax you even before you touch the drug. This is how these chains can be built up.

What is at work here is the ability of the higher nervous centres to override the lower. Often a headache can disappear because the person's attention is distracted by something that is more pressing, more urgent. Attending to it literally dismantles the previous pain pattern. Headache disappears and a new process of organisation takes over. A somewhat similar phenomenon can account for the preference of one tablet to another. More of this later.

There are some distracting activities which definitely do not ease a tension headache. So, if you've just taken a tablet, don't go jogging, don't make love, don't watch a three hour movie, don't in fact do anything that may involve the very muscles (in the eyes, face, head or neck) that you're supposed to be resting. Remember, the central nervous disorder is one of *organisation*, not of a specific thing. When you rest, you rest a specific *organisation* (higher, lower nerve functions and the personality) and this is why sleep is so effective – you rest your headache organisation.

Some people are very naïve about drugs. Pain killers operate by damping down the reception of pain impulses in the *thalamus* which is the part of higher brain functioning that distributes pain information for decisions and actions. But the *thalamus* is so much an integral part of higher brain functioning that it can ignore the pain-killing message if there isn't peace and quiet above it. So you have to help the drug to do its work. A little thought will make you realise therefore how important it is to boost the pain killer by lowering your level of activity. Also remember, depending on *how* you take the drug, the effects can take up to 20-30 minutes to work. Give the drugs time. And, once they are at work and you begin to feel better, don't presume you *are* better and rush out to carry on where you left off. Drugs wear off fairly quickly and very quickly if you exert or push things. For most people sleep is still the only thing that really clears up all the aspects of headache – even if pain killers work for you. So take the drug, slow down and get to sleep early. That is the most likely way for it to work properly for you.

There's nothing wrong with taking pain killers. They help you and they don't do any harm. But you must always bear in mind that they are designed for the 'relief' of pain. They don't claim to be pain removers nor do they stop you from getting headache. No medicine should be used beyond its stated limits and, unfortunately, this is what many people do. Got a headache? – take a pill. The only headache that this can be safely and routinely used on is if you get a very infrequent one. When you have headache often and I mean by that one or more a month, think about doing something else about it. We'll discuss just what as we go along.

Frequent or chronic tension headache
The tendency to take more pills more often increases as headaches become more frequent or don't respond to the first set of tablets you try. Quite naturally the risk of overdosing (both of variety and quantity) escalates. I have found some patients obeying the warnings on the boxes of their analgesics but taking two or three different sets, assuming that the warning about overdose only applies to the use of a particular pill. Drug effects accumulate and any sensible person should know that you have to work out your overdose level in terms of how many tablets you take in any period of time. Taking a safe dose one day is one thing; taking the same dose for four or five days in a row is another. Your body needs to recover from headache and from the pills.

The point is a simple one. Headache is a warning. You can ignore it on some occasions, especially if they are clear-cut and infrequent. To ignore recurrent or chronic headache is foolish. Taking pain killers habitually is to ignore headpain. All you are doing is reducing the pain, not attending to the signal. Moreover, you have created a second problem out of the first: chronic use of pain killers.

Now, what can you do? At the simple level, you can try

sedatives to make you more relaxed in general and this is what many people do. So long as the quantity of pain killers is reduced and not added to your consumption on top of the sedative, this is probably of some assistance in the short term. Minor tranquillisers like *diazepam* (valium) and *chlordiaze-poxide* (librium) can calm you down and make you view life with less tension than you usually do because they tend to slow down the activity of your central nervous system as a whole. Major tranquillisers simply slow down the process more and are usually used on a more permanent basis. Certain anti-depressant drugs such as *amitriptyline* (elavil) and *imipramine* (tofranil) are also prescribed in cases where depression and headache run together.

Let's be clear, however, about what precisely these drugs do. At best, they act like cotton wool, insulating and protecting the person from both the environment and their own internal discomforts such as muscle tension and headache. So long as you are on the drug, you won't feel too troubled by the things that usually distress you. However, *note* the following:

1) Being on a tranquilliser or anti-depressant does not improve the individual's capacity to organise his or her central nervous system. No learning takes place and no structural change occurs. When you stop the pills, you start the whole sequence again. Your basic organisation remains the same, assuming there has been no change in your social and personal environment. Of course, if your mother-in-law or boss who helped you to get headache has since moved to Vladivostock, you might be headache free and attribute it to the drug you took. Likewise if you won the pools.

2) Many major tranquillisers and anti-depressants have unpleasant side-effects that require other drugs to suppress them. Even mild sedatives can affect some people unfavourably.

3) Long-term use of tranquillisers is not to be encouraged. In some cases and with certain drugs, the effects of prolonged use can be dangerous (Crane, 1975). Drugs like these should only be used for chronic headache and for fairly brief periods,

otherwise you really are jumping out of the frying pan into the fire.

Okay, you suffer from chronic headache and you want to stop and you've heeded the warnings about ignoring the signals and overuse of drugs. Now what? Well, until quite recently, you had a very limited range of options. You could try psychotherapy, for example, including psychoanalysis and its derivatives; you could take posture lessons in the hope that an improved walk and comportment would ease the muscle tension. Some people have used massage, physiotherapy and physical manipulation of various muscle groups. Whether or not these options work depends on you and what you put into them. By and large, though, relief is temporary and often results in your establishing a dependency on the service which, while in some respects may be preferable to a drug dependence, may not meet your family's approval. An aspirin is one thing, an attractive masseuse or gym instructor quite another. I have known people who have tried these non-drug treatments rather over-enthusiastically end up using hot packs around the back of the neck or cold towels over the forehead. Apparently they're safer.

Things have changed a little in more recent times. Possibly because people have become more used to trends in philosophy, especially Eastern philosophy, but more likely because contemporary medicine hasn't focused enough on the common headache, so new and unusual techniques have been tried with some enthusiasm. Transcendental meditation, yoga, acupuncture and hypnosis are now considered respectable enough to find their way into medical text books.

These techniques are all founded on theories of bodily functioning that are not yet fully explored or investigated. Acupuncture, for example, operates on the premise that pain can be relieved, if not eliminated, by placing needles into key nerve points all over the body. Since we don't fully understand the mechanisms of pain anyway and it does seem to have some effect, it may work for headache sufferers. Hypnosis isn't based on any physical reactions, but is a means of controlling or influencing the minds of certain, select people. The method works through the power of suggestion that the hypnotist is able to exert over his patient. Once 'under', or in a state of semi-consciousness, the patient is then instructed to relax or to avoid the area of tension likely to produce headaches. Alternatively, the semi-conscious patient is given confidence by assertive suggestions and then sent home to practise them. Constant contact with the hypnotist and recurrent periods 'under' help to cement the hypnotic suggestions.

Yoga and meditation are fairly closely related methods involving concepts of peace of mind and bodily control based on certain Eastern philosophies of India, China and Japan. Yoga focuses on exercises, diet and attitudes of mind all being linked in an attempt to get the body and mind of the person to operate in an easy, relaxed and flowing unity. Meditation has a similar aim but achieves it by making more use of the mind's control over the body. As far as headache goes, it would seem that yoga would have the most to offer to people who are not easily able to take abstract notions and convert them into bodily relaxation. Transcendental meditation helps people to sustain their relaxation and possibly a combination of the two would do far more than each alone.

In a recent review (1978), Lance examined various studies and noted that hypnosis appeared to be more effective than transcendental meditation. Certain aspects of yoga help relieve headache (standing on your head, for example) and the benefits of acupuncture, according to Lance, seem to recede once treatment has stopped. One can expect transcendental meditation and yoga to help since they appear to improve your overall mental capacity, but before you switch to hypnosis because it is reputed to do more for your headache remember that hypnosis only works on highly suggestible people. Headache research reports that the effects of hypnosis on unhypnotisable people are non-existent, so you might not qualify.

Yoga and transcendental meditation both seek to improve your ability to relax and much the same aim is embodied in the new behaviour therapies. Growing out of psychotherapy, they appear, in my opinion, to offer the most hope for the future. Unlike traditional psychotherapy, they have focused on the specific problem to be treated and not on the patient's overall personality. Let's therefore review them briefly here.

Yoga, psychoanalysis, transcendental meditation and psychotherapy work for people who can take the *concepts* of relaxation and anxiety reduction that are involved and translate them into *actual* material changes in their personal and neural systems. Few people have either this ability or the patience to undergo what can be years of endeavour – not to mention the cost. Bear in mind, too, that people who get chronic headache don't usually make good subjects for insight learning.

The various behavioural techniques that have been developed are designed to help you bridge this gap by actually showing you how to relax and become less tense. They aren't very strong on philosophy but they are practical. Many of the techniques used have grown out of the need to help partially or fully-paralysed people, victims of stroke, cerebral palsy, accidents and so on. This has required the development of very sensitive measuring instruments and knowledge about the finer points of *autonomic* nervous system functioning. For a long time it was believed that you could not change or interfere with the *autonomic* nervous system, that it operated independently of your voluntary control (that is, you couldn't change your heart beat, your muscle tone, at will). Thanks, however, to a gentleman called Neal Miller (1969), this proposition has been much modified and now it is possible to control certain aspects of your autonomic functioning. Here's how:

Biofeedback training is a very simple, easy-to-achieve and relatively inexpensive training that you can receive at your local hospital, provided it has the staff and facilities. You sit wired up to an electromyograph (EMG) which simply measures the level of muscle activity in your head and neck muscles (doesn't hurt – promise) and records them in some convenient way. Usually they use an auditory display so that you hear a variety of sounds according to how high the activity

7

is but visual graphs (paper and pencil or oscillographs) can be used. Then they show you how to control the sound or graph to keep your activity low (relax here, relax there, think nice thoughts, etc.). If you're good, they say nice things about you which of course is the best medicine for headache sufferers. After that, it's up to you. You go home and practise and when you think you've got it (that you know *how* to lower the activity at will without the electromyograph to help you), you try to apply the learning during a headache attack or when you feel one is on the way. The training takes as little as a week and depends on you and the doctor involved. The more training the better, say some people (especially sufferers) but why this is so we will come to soon.

Relaxation training. This is very similar to EMG feedback but doesn't usually involve an EMG and is less specific. You see a therapist (it can be a doctor, psychiatrist, psychologist, social worker or even what the Americans call a behavioural engineer) and, over a few weeks or months, you learn all about your muscle groups and how to tense and relax them systematically, both singly and in groups. The idea is that you use this relaxation to ease the tension during a headache attack. So if you see someone on the bus alternately tensing and easing his muscles as discreetly as possible, you'll now know they've got a headache.

Avoidance learning. Some doctors believe it is better to avoid trouble rather than get headache. This may seem to be a rather cowardly approach to headache but for some chronic sufferers, it is the only thing that works. What happens is that you and your therapist figure out, by a systematic examination and recording of your headache pattern, the precise environmental or personal situations or stimuli which either start the headache or make it worse. Then you avoid or minimise your contact with those stimuli. Not as easy, incidentally, to do as one might think at first. Many headache sufferers are often quite ignorant as to what precisely triggers off their attacks and only a careful examination shows it up. In one woman I treated, the analysis showed that contact with her young son always triggered off a bad headache, yet she refused to accept this despite the data and the fact that everyone else in the house 'just knew' it was the relationship between them.

Cognitive retraining. A nice label this, and it describes the technique that is the reverse of the above. First, you find the psychological and environmental triggers and then you re-shape the way you react, so you don't let the headache happen. Instead of being cowed by the drug store owner or the grocer, you go in there like Atilla the Hun on the principle that a blood bath is better than a headache. Seriously, though, the therapist trains you to cope with situations that cause stress. You practise more assertive behaviour, more forceful actions, more self-confident thinking and so on.

Sound promising, don't they? But, as usual, we have to evaluate these new techniques as carefully as the old ones. One of the problems with these techniques is that no one is yet sure whether it is the technique itself or the special interest you get while you're being trained that does the work. In the last chapter, we talked a lot about the child as it develops migraine and how a lot of primary signs of distress are ignored by parents. Well, attention of any kind obviously affects the child's suffering and this is precisely what happens in adults too, although it is not nearly so effective a boost in grown-ups as it is in children. The other point to bear in mind is that *hope* in all individuals is an enormous determiner of emotional status. Some *medical* patients recover from quite serious ill-nesses after all medical intervention has failed to help, simply by having faith or hope or a drive to get well. There is nothing mystical about this. The morale of a person is directly related to the *limbic* system of the brain and from there on down.

Any new treatment creates hope and you can rise to new levels of behaviour just by expecting things to get better quickly. This is certainly true of new drugs but it is even more true of new behaviour or psychological techniques because the contact with the therapist is usually longer and both of you are as eager as each other to make it work. Unfortunately, doctors, psychiatrists and psychologists are also human and they too have careers and reputations they would like to see boosted. Far too many of the new techniques have been enthusiastically proclaimed and very favourable reports made of their effectiveness on what, from both an academic and clinical point of view, are often embarrassingly weak assessment and follow-up conditions. Very few reports check on the following:

a) How the patient copes long after all contact (at least six months) with the therapist has ceased. An uninvolved researcher should always check the results – not the original therapist.

b) How serious the condition was in the first place. Some of the studies are patients or subjects who sound completely reasonable, normal and ordinary people quite unlike the chronic headache sufferers GPs or clinicians see. These people are angry, depressed, irritable and lethargic and often very unco-operative.

c) How the patient's friends or family feel about the patient's progress and the effectiveness of the new method. Subjects frequently want to help the researcher or therapist to the extent of denying even to themselves some of the bad effects. Checking with relatives is often the only way of finding out the truth.

Some of the follow-ups cited in the research reports have taken three or four months, one took three weeks (from beginning of treatment to pronouncement of cure!) and a few took a year or more. No one can pronounce on a treatment method on this kind of basis. Speaking as an 'insider', I also must tell you that how some researchers do their follow-ups is quite unbelievable. One eminent researcher I knew was out walking and saw on the other side of a busy street one of his patients. 'How are you?' the doctor shouted across the roar of traffic. 'Fine,' was the reply and the two walked on. Yet this 'assessment' found its way into the doctor's research statistics. So be warned.

The problem with behavioural techniques is that although they are definitely headed in the right direction, teaching people how to unlearn their headache organisation, they are too peripheral. You can teach a person to relax or to control his level of muscular activity but, as we so carefully established in Chapter 8, this is only part of the complex personal and neural organisation that determines headache. Individuals can't *hold* these new developments without a systematic re-working of their entire nervous and personality pattern. Even if a patient had the continual support of a headache therapist, as time progresses the headache pattern will gradually creep back. Higher nervous functions can in time override the new learning, just as they did earlier on to form headache.

When considering the available techniques it is crucial to remember just how effective and powerful the headache organisation in the body is. It is usually established over years of practice and has whole chains of behaviour connected to it to ensure it maintains its organisation. The more chronic a condition, the more this is true. Headache is an organisation of the human body – not a specific thing like muscle tension. So I am afraid that at the moment the new techniques still have a way to go. I think they will work in mild to moderate sufferers and for a time in chronic sufferers or in chronics who are susceptible to suggestion. But, as with drugs, dependency is an important factor; remove the therapist and wait a while and things will probably return to normal. Unlike drugs, though, the techniques are seldom open to abuse and there is no risk of overdose. But again, like the attractive masseuse, there are other side-effects that are not clearly seen. The techniques do neglect the personal side of the patient's life and I have known more than one patient abandon their treatment because the family don't like their new assertive mum or dad.

Having said all that, I still believe that the future for these techniques looks encouraging. Already researchers have discovered that combining techniques into complex treatment packages is better than simply giving one alone. So you get, for example, biofeedback plus relaxation plus assertive training being offered. It works better because it tackles a more complex part of the organisational deficit. Common sense really, isn't it? As a cure, though, even combinations are open to many of the failings of the single techniques.

Before we go on to migraine treatments, we must discuss psychotherapy and psychoanalysis as possible treatment options because so many people do try them. On the face of what we have said so far, it would seem that if any discipline is going to be able to cope with a complex disorder like tension head-ache it surely would be psychotherapy. No other discipline treats the person in his social and personal context and since many psychotherapists are also medical doctors, one would have thought it was the perfect combination. So, let us try to understand why so little has been forthcoming from this direction and what can be done about it.

The first problem is that psychotherapy may cure headache but we (speaking broadly) don't know about it. Psycho-therapists are very vague in what they say they do and to understand psychoanalysts, you need to be familiar with their own special language. Even if you know what they are talking about, it doesn't always help. For one thing, they are often unwilling to conduct ordinary assessment procedures – you have to take their word for what conclusions they say they have reached. Since, as we've seen, even the word of more objective researchers has to be treated with a healthy pinch of scepticism, this is a rather dodgy state of affairs – especially if you want to duplicate their procedures. The second point is this. Psycho-therapy was originally developed for use on normal or neurotic patients where I think it is very effective. But psychotherapists have tried to apply the same principles to every other kind of disorder, simply bending the original designs a little to suit the particular problems involved. Frankly, I think they have been lazy and this won't do. Each disturbance requires its own models and its own research as I hope, by now, should be clear from our discussions in this book.

Technically, there is no reason why psychotherapy shouldn't help. But it will have to develop models and techniques purely for headache and the specific problems involved. It has done this in other areas. I use psychotherapy, for example, in treating young schizophrenics because there is a wealth of psychotherapy research and many new formulas can be applied in this area. Psychosis was in fact out-of-bounds for psychotherapy for many years but slowly researchers have opened up the field with encouraging results. This is not the case with headache.

The benefits psychotherapy brings to headache sufferers are mainly indirect. Some aspects of psychology do tap relevant areas for headache: exploring a lack of confidence, feelings of inadequacy, generalised anxiety and so on are all relevant as too are the individual's relationship to his or her parents, siblings and friends. But these areas are big areas for every part of human functioning. Everything can be tied to these issues – neurosis, psychosis, obsessivity, personality disorder and sexual deviance – the lot. Psychotherapy can also give you helpful insights but, in my experience, headache sufferers need more than insight to shift that powerful organisation.

What is more likely to help you in the short term, whatever kind of psychotherapy you choose, is going to be the special interest and attention that the therapist gives you. I think it's true to say that one of the key factors that makes psychoanalysis so attractive an option to many people (and *holds* participants to unbelievable years of it – eleven, fourteen and twenty year treatments are not that rare) is that three or five times a week, a doctor gives you his or her undivided attention. So if it's attention you're after, you know where to look.

That completes our review of treatment for muscle-contraction headache, but it isn't the last word on self-help. After the next chapter, we'll try to put everything we've learned together and map out areas and devices that you can employ to develop your own treatment programme for your headache. Again, keep an open mind. There really is a lot that a little ingenuity, a little creativity can do.

CHAPTER TEN

Treatment 2: Migraine

As one might expect, migraine has received by far the most attention and there are a number of different treatments available, ranging from the pharmaceutical to the psychological. In the practice of treatment, there is little differentiation between the five types of migraine, with the possible exception of cluster headache, so we will review the options *en masse*. Since isolated instances of migraine attack are relatively uncommon, we shall distinguish between the treatment offered once an attack has started (*symptomatic* treatment) and treatment designed to stop attacks occurring (*prophylactic* treatment).

Symptomatic treatment options
The easiest and most convenient way to intervene at this level is to take one of the pain killers we discussed for tension headache. The difficulty is that migraine is a powerful disturbance and ordinary pain killers tend not to work too well. It's a little like trying to stop a steamroller with a cricket bat. So you have to use something a little stronger and that usually means a drug which contains *ergotamine tartrate*. Analgesics work in the *thalamus* region, not near the actual site or cause of the pain, so one needs a drug to alter the state of the swollen blood vessels which are doing the damage. *Ergotamine tartrate* is such an agent. Neither a tranquilliser nor a pain killer, its major action is to constrict the blood vessels. This is a job it does very well and this is why it is preferred to other constrictor drugs. However, there are other things *ergotamine* does.

In its natural state it is a poison. Leave rye to get mouldy,

104

then bake it into bread and eat it and you will taste St Anthony's fire. Aptly named, it produces an incredible burning pain in the arms and legs which eventually become black and gangrenous. Need I add that they also fall off to induce you not to try this particular trip. And talking of trips . . . *ergotamine* is an alkaloid based on *lysergic acid* one of whose other forms is *lysergic acid diethylamide* (LSD). Like other poisons, though, *ergotamine* has its uses when controlled carefully and taken in small quantities. *Ergotamine* is used for example after childbirth to help the uterus contract but its main use is in the treatment of migraine. *Methysergide* (Deseril or Sansert) is another derivative of *lysergic acid* and it, too, is used in migraine treatment but not in acute treatments. It is less powerful than *ergotamine tartrate* and has fewer side-effects. We will come to it later.

Take *ergotamine tartrate* in one of its many forms just as the first signs start (the head pain, the first symptoms or if you just know you're in for an attack) and you should find at least some relief from the head pain that follows. It won't stop the attack altogether, nor will it stop the pain completely, although some people claim it does. By and large, it cuts down the level of discomfort and if it does that, well and good. Clinical research trials, however, have created some controversy, since *ergotamine* has not yet been shown to be more effective than placebo. In other words when people are given a harmless, ineffective drug and told it is *ergotamine*, they do about as well as if the drug really was *ergotamine*. Devious people, these researchers, aren't they? But given our discussion in the last chapter about the role of suggestibility and emotions in changing bodily functions, they have pointed to an intriguing mystery.

These kinds of personal and psychological factors may also play a role in the personal preferences people have for the various ways *ergotamine* can be taken. It is available in tablet form, combined with various other drugs like caffeine to help your body absorb the drug. You can also get it as a suppository, it can be injected, or you can get it in an aerosol can as an inhaler. There are other factors, though, that determine the method employed. Diarrhoea in the acute phase makes suppositories redundant and vomiting does the same to tablets. Working with your doctor can sort out this kind of difficulty.

Ergotamine is the most effective drug available to muscle aside migraine but its effectiveness is paid for in the dangers of its use and the difficulties involved in keeping to the thin line between overdose and helpful dose. *Ergotamine* has a double edge to it when taken in too great or too frequent quantities. In the early parts of the attack when your blood vessels are swollen, it constricts them to their normal size but at other times it can change sides and can do the reverse. Take it when you don't need it or take too much and you could actually get or prolong a severe headache. It also has sideeffects, such as creating nausea and vomiting when taken in even quite small quantities. Since migraine is a trigger-like phenomenon (one thing leads to another) that is sometimes all you need to get the migraine organisation going. Some people who swear by the stuff often get themselves into messy psychological and physical cycles that may require hospitalisation to cure. They take *ergotamine* at the first sign of trouble, then more when things don't improve quickly enough. The fresh lot brings temporary relief and then the pain starts again, only worse – and the cycle goes on. Other people become acutely dependent on the drug and I believe that many cases of *migraine status* (virtually unceasing chronic migraine) arise out of a combination of these two factors. The thing to remember, therefore, is that *ergotamine* is only useful in the early phases of migraine. Don't use it when all the symptoms are there because it can make matters worse and you could be in trouble.

Some of the other side-effects of *ergotamine* apart from the above are tingling in the hands and feet, numbness, cramps, dizziness, diarrhoea, *tachycardia*, *bradycardia* and a number of other problems. It shouldn't be used in pregnancy or if you have certain kinds of vascular and heart diseases, hypertension or certain liver and kidney diseases. So definitely make sure you co-operate very closely with your doctor when you use this drug or its derivatives.

Apart from anything else, there are new products coming on to the market all the time so that your doctor can prescribe a particular form and mixture of *ergotamine* that is best for you. Some, for example, contain an anti-emetic to help reduce nausea. He or she can also help you if you have a bad attack and you have left it too late to take *ergotamine* by giving you injections of *diazepam* (valium) or *prochlorperazine* (stematil) to help.

What do you do if you don't use *ergotamine*? Well, there are a range of other vaso-constricting drugs you can try, such as *caffeine, ephedrine, amphetamine* and the *amine, epinephrine*. None are as effective as *ergotamine* and several have troublesome side-effects of their own. The *amphetamine* story is quite well known. *Caffeine* keeps some people awake which is more serious in migraine than it sounds because sleep is still the most restorative factor. If you don't sleep, you can have problems. Most people try to lie down or to sleep with migraine as the best way of coping with the distress and alertness is the last thing they need. *Ephedrine* (a famous alkaloid used in Chinese medicine) has a similar side-effect.

Then there are other techniques that can help to a certain extent but which have obvious limitations. If you press the external *carotid* artery in your head, you may get temporary relief, especially if you do it early on when symptoms start. But don't overdo it. One person I know passed out when her husband was 'helpfully' pressing this artery. Being an absent-minded kind of fellow, he simply forgot to let go. Well, that was his story anyway. Get your doctor to *show* you where the *carotids* are.

Another interesting trick is to breathe a mixture of 10 per cent carbon dioxide and 90 per cent oxygen. It is very effective in reducing symptoms leading up to migraine. Some people apply ice-caps but they appear to be of limited value in all but the lightest of headaches.

What all these methods do is to act on the blood vessels in

an attempt to constrict them in one way or another and so prevent the onset of extreme head pain. In the late 1960s, a female volunteer at the Menninger Foundation at Topeka, Kansas, in the United States accidentally discovered that she could do much the same thing as the vein-constricting drugs simply by increasing the temperature in her hands compared to that on her forehead. She was taking part in a biofeedback research project and in the process of learning to control her hand temperature (just as we described for the muscle-contraction treatment) had a migraine which stopped after a few minutes. The discovery was researched and since then there has been quite a series of reports on this technique which are worth considering.

Basically the patient is taught to control temperature at various sites (hands, feet, forehead) by using a recording machine and learning what reactions or physical activities increase temperature. Quite simply, it is apparently relatively easy to will your hands, for instance, to get warm and this act increases the blood supply to the extremities. The originators of this technique (Sargent *et al*, 1972) aren't too clear about why it works but they report considerable success in their own clinics. It's another example of the new behavioural technology.

Most likely, if the hand-warming is doing the trick (and not suggestion or the attention shown) it is because it alters the organisation of the person's vaso-constriction network so that the blood vessels in the head reduce their circumference. I suspect though that the *act* of concentrating on a specific task for which approval and the sense of achieving something are forthcoming may distract the person's overall level of central nervous system organisation as well.

It's difficult to assess this technique because very little proper assessment has been done and it is still very new. Of interest is the fact that most of the subjects involved in the Menninger study were volunteers who had tried other treatment methods without luck and therefore they constitute a rather special group of people. Significantly, they also found it hard to get the hand-warming technique working if the headache had already set in, again demonstrating the need to act quickly. Personally, I think that this technique won't go very far as it stands. Its application is too limited. It is far more likely that the *idea* of bio-control will work far better when the sufferer is taught whole systems of counteractions and not just one or two. Friar and Beatty (1976), for example, have found that teaching people vaso-constriction techniques on the forehead (learning to control arterial pulse rates) is more useful than the same method applied to other parts of the body.* This may be due to the obvious psychological and thus central nervous system benefits to be gained from working at the site of pain rather than elsewhere. Imagine what results could be produced by doing a whole series of these training tasks.

And this is just what some investigators have discovered, although to my knowledge it hasn't been studied properly yet. Getting angry meets a number of interesting psychological requirements for the treatment of migraine. Apart from diverting attention away from the migraine, it also can be (if properly based) a powerful organisation on its own and can succeed in turning about the migraine chain. People have been reported to have stopped migraine attacks by getting furiously angry and at least one clinician has reported that you can get more out of this way of – for want of a better word – attack, than many others. Dengrove (1968) let his patients get angry and even showed them how – with fascinating results. More of this later.

That's more or less it, as far as symptomatic treatment goes. I think the choice is very limited and a great deal of research needs to be done in this area given the problems and limitations of *ergotamine*. Unfortunately, as things stand at present, I know of few researchers who are focusing on this, mainly because of the wide-spread use of *ergotamine* and because of the overriding and understandable interest in prophylactics – trying to stop attacks in the first place.

* The effects of this technique on headache was assessed incidentally by a 30-day follow-up – nearly an all-time low for follow-ups.

Prophylactic treatment options

When one begins to look at how migraine could be completely eliminated, one naturally thinks of what drugs could be taken to regulate the frequency of attacks. Most of the work on migraine has been along these lines.

The first line of attack usually employed is to take a *lysergic acid* derivative called *methysergide* on a routine basis and not tied to your actual attacks. The action of methysergide (Sansert in America and Deseril in Britain) is not fully understood. It reduces inflammation and improves the health of blood vessels and has an anti-histamine effect, all of which help avoid migraine. You take it under medical supervision on a daily basis for about six months, have a month off and then six months on, up to a maximum of eighteen months (Rawson and Liversedge, 1975). Many people claim that it works for them but some doctors are less enthusiastic about its abilities (Thrush, 1978). In any case, it does not prevent migraine attacks in all those who take it.

The dangers with this drug are somewhat less than with *ergotamine tartrate* but are nevertheless severe. It can cause skin rashes, cramps, nausea, increase in weight, vomiting, hallucinations and more seriously, fibrosis in the heart, abdomen and lungs. It shouldn't be used in children, in pregnancy, if you have vascular disease, high blood pressure, peptic ulcers or kidney or liver dysfunction. Again, it doesn't take much to constitute an overdose and most doctors agree that it shouldn't be used for too long periods and the body must be rested from it. Sometimes stopping the drug also causes a follow-up headache.

There are other drugs that are used in the prophylactic treatment of migraine, some of them with less severe side-effects and these are worth considering. *Methysergide* is a rather strong *serotonin* antagonist (serotonin plays an important role in keeping blood vessels healthy). Milder drugs with similar but weaker effects, and therefore weaker side-effects, are *Cyprohept adine hydrochloride* (*periactin*) and BC 105 (*pizotifen, sanomigran*). Both of them reduce histamine which is also a contributor to migraine attacks. Side-effects are drowsiness, increased appetite, dizziness, nausea and a tendency to make your face flush. The research findings on these drugs are favourable so far but again, follow-ups have been too short to be able to make any conclusive judgements.

Promethazine (*phenergan*) is another drug with an antihistamine property that seems to have benefited some people. It is a 'hypnotic', however, and is best taken at night. Mathews (1970) and Thrush (1978) have both reported favourably on its usefulness with children and adolescents.

Some doctors feel that migraine, like tension headache, is best controlled by making the person more tranquil in their daily lives. *Psychotropic* drugs such as *prochlorperazine* (*stemetil* or *compazine*) or the anti-depressants *imipramine* (*Tofranil*), *amitriptyline* (*Elavil*) or *trimipramine* (*surmontil*) appear to help some people and not others.

Another line of approach has been to use *Beta-blocking* drugs which act by reducing the level of blood-flow activity. This obviously reduces the pressure in swollen arteries which cause head pain. *Propranalol* (*Inderal*) is one such example.

There are many other drugs, some for specific types of migraine, some for general use. What we have described above are the major types in current use. Much work remains to be done even on those, so one has to tread carefully. You are taking fairly potent medication and we don't yet fully understand its limitations. In many instances, what the drug actually does in relation to migraine is hypothetical. We don't know the mechanisms of migraine but we know that specific drugs give some relief in some people. Hypotheses are therefore used to link the two – hence the variety of drugs and the variety of biochemical theories that you hear. None as yet is entirely right and the same goes for the drugs. Bearing that in mind, we can continue by considering some of the specific drugs for specific conditions.

Basilar artery migraine or 'menstrual' migraine is treated in some women prophylactically by using hormones such as progesterone. Despite its possible role in disrupting your monthly

111

period and its tendency to cause acne, it is better than having your uterus or ovaries removed, a practice that has only recently stopped. The argument for the surgery, incidentally, was that migraine is a disease of the endocrine glands. Whether or not hormones are a significant cause in this kind of migraine is still under debate, so don't expect too much.

A newish drug called *Clonidine* (a *noradrenaline antagonist*) has been used in general without startling results but appears to have some value in treating people who are prone to triggering off their attacks by eating certain foods. But some of its side-effects may not make it worth your while trying. They include drowsiness, dry mouth, itchiness and depression.

Cluster headaches have responded to the use of *lithium carbonicum (Polfa)* according to several researchers including a Polish team in Lodz (Klimek *et al*, 1979). *Lithium*, originally used in the treatment of gout, then as a sedative and anti-convulsant, then in heart patients (with unfortunate results), found its way into psychiatry where it is used as the bedrock treatment of mania in manic-depressive patients (Klein and Davis, 1969). Now it may help cluster headache sufferers. I give you the history to give you some idea of the kind of thing that happens to a drug or to combinations of drugs as research goes on and to help you realise that no one drug is just one thing: it is far more complex. The Polish authors note, incidentally, that its use in the treatment of chronic cluster headache may be limited.

Like tension headache, drugs and other interventions are probably best used in combinations in the treatment of migraine and this seems to be the general direction research is following. The new drugs have bits and pieces of everything, hoping that a particular combination works for you. Thus you can get anti-nausea bits, tranquillising bits, bits to help your body absorb the pain killer and so on.

Overall, there is a pretty wide choice allowing most conditions of migraine to be helped at least in part, and for a time. In really extreme and chronic cases, you can go to hospital where all sorts of more effective things can be done for a limited time. For example, you can be anaesthetised if you can't sleep, you can be heavily tranquillised, you can be *heparinised* (using an anti-coagulant that stops headache), you can even have surgery, and so on. Then, gradually, you can be helped to recovery.

The drawback to all these procedures is that you can't stay on medication of any kind forever. Without medication, as we pointed out earlier, you are back to normal. No learning actually takes place. Further, some people can't take the drugs involved because they have other ailments that prevent it. What do they do and what do you do if you don't want to use drugs for treatment?

You could try surgery, though by and large this is not very favourably viewed by many family doctors. Knight (1968) describes the techniques employed (*sypathectomy*) and describes how useful they can be in some cases. He notes, however, that there must be a fairly well-defined area of migraine (unilateral and always the same side) before surgery can be considered. Since we know so little about the cause of migraine, it seems to me to be a fairly extreme thing to undertake. I know of people who have had surgery for headache and found little changed afterwards – same old migraine, same old frequency. Until we know more, I would say it has only to be used as a last resort.

You could try glasses. For a long time it was believed that eyestrain was related to migraine and a good many adolescents I know were given glasses for near-perfect vision as a way of reducing their pain. But most doctors now think that this is not the case (Cocklin, 1978) and I think they are probably right, since wearing spectacles won't change the migraine pattern. However, the relationship of the way you look at things, between eyestrain and the structure of migraine, is quite complex. We will discuss this further in the next chapter, so don't dismiss this aspect altogether.

The idea of wearing glasses to help with migraine is not so strange as it sounds. Wearing dark glasses does seem to help some people at least avoid bright lights. This leads us to the next general option for avoiding migraine. You can keep clear of the things that seem to or are likely to precipitate an attack. After drugs, this trigger theory of therapy is the most common.

The theory is simple. Find out what causes you to develop migraine and then avoid it. Under this heading falls a whole range of topics from diet to certain weather conditions*, from bright lights, certain smells (tobacco smoke in a crowded bus, for example) to too much television, from over-exertion to getting up late. The British Migraine Trust publish a pamphlet called *Understanding Migraine* (London, 1979) containing all these and it is worth having a look at. It might give you some clues as to what to look for.

What you must do to find out if there are in fact certain things that cause or seem to bring on your migraine is to examine each possibility carefully. Don't go through a long list. Pick the ones that seem to apply to you. If lights, for example, have never worried you, don't waste your time on them. Start by keeping a record of each of your migraine attacks and see if you were in the same place or under the same set of conditions for each attack. If you were in a bus *and* people were smoking, put it down and then next time see if being on a bus but moving into the no-smoking section still gives you a headache. If it doesn't, then smoking is your problem. To be certain, you would have to keep recording events to discover exactly what is at the root of the cause. Motion, for example, can often cause migraine under certain conditions, but not others. If a migraine sufferer is on a crowded bus, irrespective of smoke, he might be upset because he can't see where the bus is going. This, together with the smoke, seems to bring on a migraine attack.

By careful trial and error you can often pin-point which conditions to avoid. A little thought can help you identify complex patterns of events which are more often than not

* No one knows if Britain's appalling weather is the major cause of migraine. It is believed, however, that certain tribes in Africa never suffer from migraine. Perhaps it's all that sun.

found to be the cause of migraine attacks. What is it about smoke, for example, that upsets you? Is it the smell, or the irritable effect on your breathing? Or do you just feel suffocated? There's smoke and smoke. Some migraine sufferers hate tobacco smoke but are quite happy about wood or engine smoke, so why the link? Some people think that tobacco smoke is one of several stimuli that have negative connotations for certain people. Smoke, certain foods, wines, certain lights, certain movements, may have been associated in the person's past with unpleasant situations or memories that became in time linked to the migraine pattern.

By the time most migraine sufferers are in their twenties they have established their specific cause pattern. But they should try to explore their thinking further both to help them reduce their discomfort by trying to avoid the painful stimulation and by building on the discoveries they have already made.

Only one kind of thing may cause your migraine to start, but looking through the list, one can see that the triggers are things which are often quite *hard* to avoid. How can you avoid, for example, the bright glare of sunlight suddenly hitting your eyes from a car's windscreen? You can avoid certain foods but if you have several triggers, you could well tend to organise your evasive action so much that simply going for a walk becomes torture. The day when migraine sufferers are easily identified by their dark glasses, scarves, ear plugs and slow walk may not be far off.

The point is that triggers are valuable self-diagnostic tools which again only work for some people. To avoid the triggers is, in my opinion, of only limited value. Having gone to the trouble of finding them, why not *use* them to research your own condition? More of this in the next chapter.

All the other more elaborate methods of intervention we discussed in the last chapter, such as yoga, psychotherapy, transcendental meditation and so on, have a bearing on migraine. We could argue that they apply as general helpers because, despite the differences between muscle-contraction

115

(tension?) and migraine (anxiety?) headache, these techniques are sufficiently broad-based to be able to work at both components. Further, if migraine is such an all-encompassing disorder, it could be argued that psychotherapy of all things would help. Most doctors would probably agree that no migraine treatment is complete without some form of counselling or psychotherapy to back up whatever else is used. Certainly, advice, concern, attention and bits of insight all help treatment and, of course, complicate assessment. In one report, drug-free tablets work about as well as some actual drugs, which just shows how effective some doctors' attention can be (Friedman, 1975). The trouble is, again, that there are few reports about the actual results of psychotherapy and so it's hard to specify just what can be done.

More specific reports have, however, emerged from behavioural scientists working in this area and in place of good psychotherapy studies, we'll have to settle for those.

As we noted earlier in this chapter, the biofeedback and hand-warming techniques don't really work in the prophylactic sense. This is why researchers have concentrated on three basic training programmes to help sufferers. The first, relaxation, we are familiar with from Chapter 9, and so too with the second, assertive training. The third is 'systematic desensitisation' and this may need a word of explanation. In 1958 Joseph Wolpe devised a technique called 'reciprocal inhibition'. Very briefly, a person suffering from anxiety or tension was first taught how to relax. Then he or she and the therapist constructed a tension-producing hierarchy, with very frightening things at the top and less frightening ones lower down. Patients would then start with the thing that produced the least fear and anxiety, think about it as the anxiety rose and then relax. Slowly, and by gradual exposure, step-by-step to more frightening things, the person becomes desensitised and learns to associate physical relaxation with the thing they feared.

These techniques all focus on making the patient more relaxed, more assertive and less anxious in general. This is not to be confused with specific anxieties that cause migraine.

Studies done in Australia by Mitchell and Mitchell (1971) have found that each of the techniques appears to help reduce the number of migraine attacks and that what they call 'combined desensitisation' (systematic desensitisation plus assertive training) works better than relaxation alone. Work done by Paulley and Maskell (1975) at the Ipswich Hospital in England differed in technical theory but used relaxation, group discussion sessions and psychotherapy and this also seems to have provided relief to sufferers.

What is actually doing the work remains unclear. In the interests of helping patients, it's the general direction that counts and these techniques will have to be systematically examined in time. Follow-ups in the studies have been either superficial and/or made too soon afterwards. What again is clear is that the broad offensive used in the studies seems to guarantee a more effective treatment than a single dimension applied alone.

Having presented the major types of possible interventions, it would be nice to know which are the more effective. Mitchell and Mitchell said that their methods successfully *eliminated* migraine in 22.2 per cent of a sample of their patients and substantially *reduced* it in 70.4 per cent. Curran *et al* (1967) reported that the drug *methysergide* as a prophylactic *eliminated* migraine in 3.1 per cent of their sample and helped another 52.1 per cent. On the surface, the behavioural techniques seem better, but bear in mind that the Mitchells' figures are for twenty-two patients, Curran's for 2,329. The Mitchells' subjects were, in the main, volunteer students or university staff, Curran's were not. What matters is that both figures for elimination are very low. When you add that to the fact that removal of the drug and the therapeutic research team would both probably produce relapse, then you see that we have a way to go in achieving a cure for migraine.

The Big Questions, as you can imagine, are what would a curative treatment look like? Where would one be found? If you want to know the answer, then simply turn the page and read the next exciting instalment ..

CHAPTER ELEVEN

Towards a Cure 1: Concepts, Diagnosis and the mild headache

First, we need an overall view of what we have found so far. One: muscle-contraction headache and migraine are the most commonly occurring types of headache. Two: all existing treatment methods help some people some of the time but not all of the people all of the time. Three: treatments aimed at one level generally are less effective than those aimed at more than one as in the desensitisation package, the analgesics-cum-anti-emetics, the combination of analgesics and tranquillisers and so on. All of these point to the complex, psychosomatic organisation of headache. Four: no treatment seems capable of continuing to work after it has been stopped. This may be a bit unfair to those people who have made full recoveries after a course of drugs or psychotherapy but since these are generally exceptions rather than the rule, the majority rule, okay? Five: there are many clues as to where a cure may lie and several fairly clear directions that need exploration.

Before exploring them, though, let's be quite clear about the notion of 'cure' we will use in this and the next chapters.

What does the word 'cure' mean? The dictionary meaning that I prefer is *restoring to health* (the Shorter Oxford, 1970). The idea of a full remedy or complete healing are ways we have of interpreting 'restoring to health' in a narrow, abstract sense. Usually, we talk of a cure in the sense of a miracle: 'Before taking "the cure" everything was terrible, now everything is fine.' It's part of the twentieth century's obsession with perfectionism. We can design and build exquisitely perfect and

118

precise material objects and we expect to see the same in human affairs. We look for a hundred per cent efficiency, thinking that to be 'normal' is to be perfectly happy, perfectly healthy, perfectly beautiful and so on.

What we forget is that a perfect machine is an artificial machine. No machine, bridge or instrument exists on its own. It is used by humans and it is this which makes it real. And it is of course here that a machine becomes less than perfect. It dates, it can deprive people of jobs, it can kill, depending on how it is used. Youn cannot separate how a thing is *used* from what it is.

The human body is a pretty efficient machine but it, too, dates, can deprive people of jobs and can kill. So what is the normal, healthy, state of the human? In far too many people's eyes, the answer to this question is abstract and ideal. Most people think proper human functioning occurs in a rational, healthy, problem-free, young human body full of all the 'right' traits such as certainty, sensitivity, intelligence and capability. So obviously, if we are going to think about a 'cure' for any human ailment like headache, we are going to have to be clear before we begin about quite what we mean by the healthy state we have as an objective and about how to get there.

This is not a pedantic issue. How we conceive of a cure is determined by the general conditions in which we live. Since we live in the twentieth century and since technology and precision are important in our lives, we tend to see a cure for headache in an absolute sense. And we tend to believe that only technology is going to get us to it. Healthy functioning for the headache sufferer means, in this view, to be completely headache-free. How is this to be achieved? Develop a tablet, something convenient and easy to take? Search for a 'quickie' cure that works the same for everyone? In other words, we need an instant 'cure' that suits one and all.

This is not how I view cure nor is it how I view the healthy functioning state of the individual to which we want the headache sufferer to return. The healthy individual is, as I said earlier, unlikely to be headache-free, nor is he likely to be problem-free. In fact, to draw several strands of argument together, I think having a chronic or frequent headache is a way of opting out of dealing with certain crucial problems in living that you have to face and deal with in order to be healthy.

Throughout the book I have given a rough theory of normality based on the individual meeting and dealing with problems at each level of biological organisation. We have talked about the problems of coping with conflict and living together, the problems of separating and becoming independent from the family, the need to become an individual and forming a proper attachment with another person and the need to develop a stable and effective pattern of brain and central nervous system activity. All these problems are related and involve each level acting in a complex way with every other. Headache is not just a central nervous system problem, nor is it a personality problem. It is a problem of human biology which means it arises out of *how* we use our bodies. Headache is a symptom that arises because the person cannot cope with problems of living and so develops head pain under the pressure. In avoiding one problem, you create another. This, I believe, is the psychological and social significance of headache and it is this that must be looked at. Successful living is not *removal* of problems, but *facing* them. At every level of biological activity, from the simplest nerve cell upwards, you will find that, without problems to continually stimulate and test them, the organism will gradually deteriorate through lack of use.

The danger with headache is that it is very easy to ignore this and to make yourself a kind of patient. It's a bit like abandoning an exercise or a game at the very first sign of stiffness or cramp, on the grounds that your mum and dad suffered cramps – it runs in the family, it's inherited, biochemical . . . all of which are used to convince yourself that you have just cause to stop playing. Headache is a sign that your body is over-stressed. It can't take it, you are frightened, you want to run away, avoid something, rest, sleep, anything – but can't. You don't need a justification for being frightened or stressed – you have a right to these things. Making a condition out of

120

headache is a bad and unhealthy way of justifying perfectly normal human responses. A cramped muscle should be rested and then re-worked – not wrapped in cotton wool and never used again.

My view of cure in headache and migraine is therefore those things which will free you from side-tracking yourself into a kind of dead-end and help you to face the real, the crucial and the important problems that make for healthy living. Having and facing the *right* problems is the aim of my 'cure' thesis, so it follows that we are not interested in *solving* these 'right' problems, but simply in taking them head-on. Thus I won't attempt here to tell you *how* to behave correctly or what you *should* be doing out there in society, but I will tell you how to get off the headache problem complex. And this leads us to the second important idea we have to be clear about.

Our twentieth-century view of cure is a general one. We think of the same cure for everyone, based on an idealised, artificial, image of the healthy individual. If, however, we accept that 'healthy' means facing problems, then it follows that what *you* do with your problems is your business. All that matters is that you are moving in the right direction. 'Cure' for you, then, is going to be your own job. You have your own specific set of problems in life, your own individuality, your own surroundings – even your very own headache pattern. Cure, then, is going to be *your* cure. All that matters for you is that you stop having headache. How you do it is up to you. No one else can do the job for you. At best we can help you with advice and point you in the right direction. The only rule is that you face the right problems.

Now you can see where you come in. You have to work at yourself to create your own hypotheses and take the steps necessary to test them out – with help and guidance as to where to look, where to begin, what to watch out for. Your cure is in your hands because your interaction with your environment has created the specific conditions for your specific headache complex. If headache was a straightforward organic illness, we wouldn't need such a complicated set of ideas to fix it and you

121

wouldn't have much to do. However, it isn't and along with a number of other psychosomatic problems, its cure requires *you*.

What I propose to do is throw out hypotheses to direct you and to set you thinking along the right lines. So follow the threads of what I'm saying and think closely about the questions asked. I don't know the answers – you do. You might not like what I have to say sometimes, but remember, the aim is to make you aware of what you are hiding or missing. Don't expect to be treated like a patient or to be nursed or to get undue sympathy – they never helped anyone face the right problems.

A headache is an organised chain of events that happens to you. If we could identify that pattern for each individual and tell each person how to change it, we would have a cure for headache. No one change alone at one level, be it social, psychological or neurological, will – on its own – alter the essential structure of an individual's headache organisation. It may modify it – but not change its basic headache-making tendency.

We are looking for a way or ways of changing the organisation. Since each person's organisation is going to be specific to him or her, the clues contained in this part of the book are general clues, hints about where to look and what to do with what you find.

Diagnosing your headache type
It is possible to identify four kinds of headache type depending on the degree to which your headaches impose upon and disrupt your normal healthy function. Have a look at the list and decide which heading you fall under.

Normal headache. This is the constructive, planned headache we spoke of earlier. It occurs infrequently and always occurs in a certain situation. You get it purely as a result of choosing clearly and rationally to put stress on yourself for some gain or other. Secondly, people who get normal headaches don't *use* them to gain sympathy or understanding. If they do, it is on

122

rare occasions only and can be clearly recognised. Finally, normal headaches are used by the person as keys to intriguing problems in personal development, not as excuses for avoiding issues. Theoretically, someone with normal headaches will find them diminishing in time as they mature and their characters develop. We won't be concerned much with this type, except to try to return people in the other three categories to it.

Mild interference headache. This is probably best described as a bloody-nuisance type of headache pattern. They come at you fairly frequently, you haven't really much idea why *you* of all people should be troubled by them but they don't seem to be very serious and they don't really incapacitate you. The trouble is, though, that once you've got it, you have to stop to take a tablet or two and this irritates you more than anything. Perhaps you wouldn't really like to think of yourself as being headache-prone and would prefer to be in the first category above. If you have any doubt, keep a careful note in your diary of when you have a headache and do this for two months. If the total exceeds two, this is your category.

Moderate interference headache. This category describes headaches that do interrupt your daily life at about or near the 50-50 level. Half the time you have a headache, the other half of your time, you don't. In this category, we include migraine headache, even if they cluster together; any combination of headache in fact which troubles you for more than a third of your time.

Chronic or major interference headache. This condition is defined by any headache pattern that interferes with your life greater than the 50-50 level. People who fall into this category most often describe their lives as being devoted to their headaches or dominated by them. Chronic muscle-contraction as well as chronic migraine headache sufferers fall into this category.

In the rest of this chapter, we will focus on the mild interference headache and in the next two, on moderate and major interference types respectively.

Mild interference headache

You get a headache or migraine and it bothers you. While it isn't a massive problem, it's got to the point where they are cropping up too often for your liking. Let's take it from there. First you need some relief. You can't work on your headache while you're in pain, so take something. Ask your doctor or your chemist for assistance here, and then, once you're free of the pain, take the trouble to sit down and do a little homework.

If you remember, earlier on we talked about the way head pain is a signal that something is wrong and that in most cases the individual systematically ignores the preceding but less obvious physical and psychological signs. In Chapter 8, on migraine people, we talked about how this systematic avoidance can become so well-organised that it interferes in both personality and central nervous system organisation (the 'frozen' development of migraine children). Now, the mild-interference headache sufferer is not going to be in such a state. He or she is going to have, by and large, a fairly normal level of physical and psychological organisation and development but in some areas there will be dysfunction. At the simplest level, the greater the dysfunction, the more interference the person suffers from headache. The task for the mild-interference sufferer is therefore to find the areas in their lives which are causing the trouble and then to take action to improve the way they cope in these areas.

One of the characteristics of people in this category is that very often they do not relate their headache to specific causes – they just 'happen' without any apparent preceding stress or warning. A headache simply arrives. In some cases, there is a kind of arbitrary analysis, such as: 'Oh yes, it must have been *that* which upset me', and the individual points to an obvious recent stress event. For these people, headaches are an irritant, unnecessary, a sign of weakness, not worth bothering about and so, consequently, they are quickly forgotten or easily pushed aside as an embarrassing irrelevancy.

People who fall into this category suffer from an under-attention to themselves and their bodies and the first line of

124

attack is to open up awareness of stress areas and bodily reaction. If, therefore, what we discuss seems commonplace to old headache hands, bear in mind that your mild sufferer is a novice at the game. To the newcomer, follow the clues discussed below, try to answer the questions and you may well help yourself on the road to recovery and not to becoming an old hand.

Clues from medication. One of the first places to start your explorations in self-awareness is to examine the drugs that you have taken for headache, especially the ones that have worked for you either in reducing the pain or in reducing the frequency of attacks. Think back: did a simple pain killer work? Or did you have to call your doctor in to prescribe something stronger? This is important. If a simple analgesic worked, the chances are that irrespective of frequency of headache, the organisation of your headache is probably fairly slight. The stronger the pain killer (both in dosage and type), the more resistant to intervention the headache is and the more firmly embedded its organisation. If you have migraine and you have to resort to *ergotamine tartrate*, then your migraine, irrespective of type, is probably fairly well embedded.

Now, did a pain killer work or did you find a tranquilliser or sedative did the trick? If you've found a successful pain killer, don't bother with a tranquilliser, but if you did find a tranquilliser helpful – either in relieving an attack or in reducing future attacks – was it a mild one or a severe one? Again, your doctor or chemist will be able to tell you which is which.

If you needed a major tranquilliser, it more than likely means that at this time you are probably under a fairly severe load of broadly-based emotional stress which may or may not be temporary, such as a death in the family, a divorce, a new job and so on. If the pattern has persisted for longer than six months, then it is quite likely that it is not temporary and your personal adjustment is not good. You will have to attend to yourself more than you perhaps realised.

If you needed a mild tranquilliser, then the chances are that

125

the headache organisation you possess is fairly likely to change and is more tied to current events than a long-term pattern in your own adjustment. This doesn't let you off the hook, it means that your day-to-day security may be placed in the wrong things.

Clues from side-effects. You've taken your normal, routine pain killer or tranquilliser – what happened? Did you have any of the usual side-effects? Like nausea, dizziness, drowsiness, bad taste in your mouth? If you did, and they were fairly moderate, that's quite normal and part of the cross we all have to bear when taking drugs. But if the side-effects virtually wiped you out, there may be a clue in there about you, as too there may be if you noticed no side-effects whatsoever. In my experience, mild-frequency headache sufferers fall into two broad reactive types when it comes to drug effects. The first is characterised by a kind of over-reaction to anything out of the ordinary – a simple side-effect upsets you out of all proportion. The second is characterised by a complete indifference to side-effects and is part of the person's general make-up.

How do you react to medicines taken in general? If you *always* ignore side-effects or have a bad time with them, irrespective of what drug you take, then your system is more unstable than you think. If you're the overreactive type, then you may be a walking disaster looking for something to trigger you off and headache is a convenient and socially-acceptable way of 'collapsing' while retaining a stiff upper lip. If you're the other type, then headache is the least of your troubles. Ask people what they think of you and you'll probably find they consider you to be a bit insensitive, unfeeling, perhaps even callous or indifferent.

Clues from your attitudes to drugs and doctors. Do you hate taking drugs? Do you hate doctors? Many people dislike drugs and doctors in about equal proportion and again therein lies a clue to general functioning. A couple of bad experiences with either drugs or doctors shouldn't make you hate them and if they do, then you should really examine the basis of your attitudes. Some people latch on to conveniently and easily identified things such as this to express pent-up frustration and anger in general. It's safer to attack them than the actual things in your life that may have caused the frustration in the first place. You may find it easier, for example, to be angry or hurt with a doctor's brusqueness or authoritarianism than with your boss's or your father's or your mother's. Likewise, you can comfortably hate the drug industry without fear of reprisals in the middle of the night from black-leather jacketed pharmaceutical manufacturers. Your anger may be due to a general feeling of fear and inhibition because you feel pressured and restricted in your social relationships.

I'm not saying necessarily that this is why you dislike doctors or drugs or, alternately, that they both are really angels and quite innocent. I'm saying that the *intensity* of your feeling should give you a valuable clue to your psychological state. You may find, for example, that you don't like seeking help, or admitting that you need help. You may resent the impersonality of drugs and some doctors and may want far more from these channels of help than they can give or you are yourself aware of. People with headache *do* have problems in admitting 'weaknesses' or seeking help. They either over-do it and flog a drug or a doctor to death out of all proportion to their real suffering or they under-do it and resent bad management like hell. It would help you to know which type you are.

Let's move on a bit now to more general clues that might emerge in your day-to-day activity unrelated to headache as such. Think about how you view yourself and how you cope with quite ordinary problems such as crowds, rush hours, how you drive, and how you think.

Clues from your general level of awareness
Someone stands on your feet in a bus or train. What is your first reaction? Do you yell or do you push them off? Are you polite and patient, or offensive and brusque? Most chronic headache sufferers are polite and long-suffering to the extent that they will not make a social fuss without the greatest of

provocations. The important clue to your level of functioning is this: how aware are you of your bodily discomfort and what do you do about it? Obviously some people are born with low or high pain threshholds, but that's not the point. What do you do when you feel pain or discomfort? Do you find that you only show it to certain people but not to others? Are you the kind of person who would be too embarrassed to scream for help, even if you were drowning?

Headache sufferers by and large hide their pain levels. It helps them to be 'special', to have a 'superior' feeling over other people who show feelings. Headache is a respectable phenomenon – much more socially tolerated than crying. Some headache sufferers are so good at hiding pain that they push themselves beyond normal limits of stress, quite unaware that they shouldn't.

Then there's a different kind of sensitivity, a more social one. Here's a check list of common areas of frustration connected to sensitivity. See if any apply to you:

1. You're standing in a queue or in a bookshop, someone stands right next to you – almost on top of you. You feel like exploding inside but you don't.

2. You shake hands with someone (male or female) and they don't know when to let go – it infuriates you.

3. Someone insists on reading your paper over your shoulder quite openly and ignores your look or wince of disapproval.

4. Someone, a friend, a child or relative, insists on hugging, kissing or touching you, any one of which makes you wince inside.

5. Dogs or cats or other animals come up to you without bidding and insist on sniffing you or jumping up. It drives you mad. Animals or children leave marks or stains on your clean clothes which infuriates you.

6. You're in a hurry and someone gets in your way – it may be in a lift, in the office, even when you're out driving. You feel like screaming or pushing them out of the way but you don't.

7. While you're trying to get something done that demands

128

patience and concentration, someone or something is making a racket but you really feel you can't ask them to be quiet.

8. Someone insists on teasing or playing or touching you when someone you want to impress is around and you're caught between wanting approval and not wanting the teaser to be hurt if you tell them to cut it out.

9. Someone is rude to you but you don't dare say anything, either because they're bigger than you, they will make a public fuss or you're scared of their power.

10. You're at a dinner party or similar function and someone is drunk and falls all over you. You feel like machine-gunning them but it jams.

Now perhaps you'll understand why earlier I said that the idea of the silent football or ice-hockey game wasn't such an unusual phenomenon. The point here is not that any one of these can cause your headache but that this list should give you a clue as to how high your general level of frustration is. If you ticked more than two items on the list, believe me, you are frustrated and you may really just be wandering around waiting for a headache to happen. If none of the items on the list applies to you, have a look at yourself during a normal day and see if there aren't perhaps very similar situations that cause frustration to build up. The essential feature you should be looking for is a general inability to reduce your level of tolerance and no suitable means of expressing yourself.

Clues from your personal relationships

If none of the above have provided clues as to where your particular problem area is then give some thought to how you relate to people. How do you view people in general? Are any of the following statements in line with your views?

1. You can't really trust people.

2. People basically are selfish and only look after their own interests.

3. This world is a tough one and you have to be tough to survive.

4. Look after number one.

5. The world is in a terrible state.

6. People are fools.

7. If only people were more like me.

8. People are weak.

9. We'd all be a lot happier if everybody was a bit more responsible and worked harder.

10. People give up too easily.

If you ticked more than one, then it is pretty likely that you may hold quite stereotyped views about people and about how people should or should not behave. A healthy person tends to look at him- or herself and at others in a very easy light, believing what people *are* is more important than what they *should* be. This doesn't mean an absence of criticism but rather that the criticism is directed at specific and clearly defined failings in people (including oneself) as they operate in society. Your criticism, if you ticked a number of the above items, is outward, general and indiscriminate, based on a general feeling of depression, impotence and perhaps even despair. You more than likely don't analyse yourself and those close to you properly and, more significantly for your headache, you probably don't express yourself as you should.

If you hold stereotyped ideas about people in general it is very likely that you behave to those around you in a stereotyped way too. That is, you are polite to 'elders and betters', you love those you are supposed to love and dislike those you are allowed to dislike etc., etc. The person doesn't matter, neither does the fact that each close relationship should be a complex mixture of a wide range of emotions: anger, love, hurt, frustration, sexuality, affection and so on. Look at this next list and see how uncomfortable any of the items make you feel:

1. I love my wife (or my husband) dearly and hate him (or her) too at odd moments.

2. I respect my boss but I would also like to kick his or her face in sometimes.

3. I wish I had never had children but I do so love them.

4. I love my father but there are times when I wish I had a different one.

130

5. I would like to frighten my wife (or husband) sometimes just for the sheer hell of it.

6. Nothing would make me more satisfied on occasions than to slap my mother's face, love her though I do.

7. You always hurt the one you love.

8. I am happily married, have a lovely wife (husband), lovely children. I have a super job, a wonderful boss, a secure future and tomorrow I'm going to run away from it all.

9. I enjoy responsibility, I feel it makes a man (or woman) out of you. It's something to feel proud about inside, makes you stand a little taller each time you face it and take it. How I wish I was irresponsible.

10. When I have a fight with someone, or a disagreement, I find I have a renewed respect for them but from then on I hate them, especially if they win.

If you found *none* of these ideas either intriguing or satisfying, then you are probably highly stereotyped and act out roles rather than enter into proper relationships. Underneath you are probably frightened of people, unconfident and, I *hate* to say this, but you probably get your kicks in secret little ways that would shock your loved ones if they knew. If this last statement angers you, don't tear the book up – examine yourself and ask why you felt so guilty or so indignant. Don't, please though, get a headache on my account. There is nothing wrong with having secret little vices or pleasures – no matter how you define them. The thing that's wrong is if you pretend *to yourself* that you don't. And that leads me on to the last point that we have room for.

Most headache sufferers tend to be very bland about their own self-assessment. When asked, they smile and blush shyly and admit to a few conventional vices and a lot of conventional nicenesses and then clam up. They really don't know themselves very well and this is because they have never been made to or seen the necessity to. Not only do they view others stereotypically but they do the same to themselves. In keeping other people at arms length, they also stop themselves from having encounters and experiences that are the food and drink of the rest of mankind and which help to unlock one's own self-awareness.

Clues from your emotional reactions
Three things are relevant here: do you have emotional reactions, do you *act* them out, and do you use them in the right place and at the right time? It's one thing to be able to cry, for example, but quite another to cry properly, that is, appropriately. First, here are two lists of emotional reactions. See how many you engage in:

List A	List B
Crying	Puffing your cheeks out
laughing	frowning
shouting	glaring
screaming	biting your nails, lips, tongue or cheek
giggling	
sighing	screwing your eyes up
whistling	scowling
singing	grating your teeth
hitting	sneering
pinching	weeping (not the same as crying)
slapping	poking
tickling	having intercourse (not the same as making love)
making love	
licking your lips	sniffing
dribbling or drooling	nodding your head a lot
desiring	lusting (not the same as desiring)
sleeping deeply	coveting
being noisy	possessing
running around	rushing around (not the same as running around)
being playful	
being angry	playing games like chess, mastermind etc
	being sarcastic
	being silently disapproving

Add up the number you ticked from each list. If you had more from list A than list B, fine. But if you were about 50-50 or had more from list B, then your emotional reactions may be muted or inappropriate. It is, however, at least established. If you ticked *nothing* at all or only one or two items from List A or you only ticked things in List B, then your reactivity is very limited and needs a lot of work. You may feel things inside but you don't act on them.

Secondly, there's the question of appropriateness. Being able to cry is a good thing but when do you cry? Only at funerals, births, weddings and on receipt of good news? Or do you cry at other times too? Crying at funerals is socially acceptable but not what we mean here by 'appropriate'. Crying when you get hurt, angry, frustrated, tired, is the kind of appropriate crying we are getting at *and* crying when you feel like it – not an hour later or when things have really built up. The same for the other emotional reactions. Suppressing a giggle may seem a harmless enough thing to do but if you also suppress a whole range of other things, you're getting close to the picture of playing football in silence. Think about it.

Putting the clues together
Not all of what we have said applies to any one person. If you get mild-interference headache, then, by definition, large parts of your functioning are fairly healthy and normal. The trick is to find the weak areas in your make-up, using these clues, and then to act on what you have found. There are, obviously, far more clues around than we've discussed here and if we've missed you out, sorry.

Now let's look at how your healthy functioning interacts with the blind spots. For a start, don't try to think of these blind spots as things you must suppress in order to cure your headache. It really is no good going round all tough and macho-like, assailing old ladies and assorted bus conductors. You can't *impose* a stereotype 'healthy' behaviour on to your personality. The thing to do is to get away from stereotypes and develop the poor parts of your functioning.

133

What I'm getting at is the fact that close examination of yourself along the lines of the clues discussed earlier, will expose a lot of things about yourself that you are really already aware of somewhere inside. In other words, the thought or impulse has crossed your mind before. You will have got tense, angry, upset, frustrated, frightened by things, have recognised it and wanted to do something about it but couldn't. This is where mild-interference headache sufferers differ from the more extreme sufferers: you have a better chance of acting on your feelings and insights because a good deal of your functioning is already alerted to the need to do so.

What you have to do now is to put together hypotheses about your own headache patterns. You have to examine yourself and your headache and try to make possible cause-and-effect chains. Use the clues and also use your instincts – little bits of ideas and impulses that come into your head even if you think they are silly or childish. In fact the more silly or childish the better – they are the most reliable signs of deeper feelings in repressed people.

Once you have a hypothetical chain, you have to test it out. Be prepared to reject it and to have to find new ones or to have to make the first one more complex or elaborate as you go along. Now let's look at some possible chains and show you how to construct them and how to test them out.

Hypothetical chains
Step One. The simplest level of chain construction would be as follows: 'I went to the supermarket and one of the cashiers was rude to me. By the time I got home, I realised I had a headache. Now that I think about it, I remember really getting cross at the time but I let it pass.' So your link would be: failure to get cross → headache. You can probably construct any number of such simple chains if you start watching your own reactions instead of brushing them off or dismissing them. Don't, however, do anything about changing your behaviour yet. You need to build up a complex web of hypotheses first. As I have said, headache is a complex phenomenon and no single

134

action will eliminate it. You must identify your headache organisation and first you need many carefully worked out hypotheses to give you an accurate cross-reference on yours – just like you need an accurate cross-reference to a point on a map.

Quite apart from this, you need practice at attending to yourself, getting used to taking time to think about your sensory input and your reactive processes. Start a headache diary, note down when you have one, what happened earlier and what your thoughts were. Above all, don't rush it – we are interested in a cure, not a quick exit without doing any work. Jot down any bits of odd information you think are relevant.

Once you have mapped out your headache pattern over a period of six to eight weeks, you should have found a fair number of different situations that seem to cause them. Don't incidentally jump to conclusions that the first hypothesis you find (failure to get cross → headache, for example) is the model for the rest. Look for other hypotheses too. This is where many people go wrong. They try to take short cuts by reducing all their causes to one simple one and it simply does not work. No one thing causes them – it is an organisation and it is unique to you.

Step Two. Probe each hypothesis carefully. Take the first one (like, failure to get angry → headache) and check to see *exactly* what happened. You can do this by going back to the supermarket and seeing what happens or by comparing other situations in which this hypothesis comes up. Perhaps it is more complex than you thought. Did the 'failure to get cross' sufferer contribute to the trauma by being too casual or too brusque to the cashier? Many chronic headache sufferers are fairly haughty and superior in their treatment of people they consider 'inferior'. Perhaps our 'un-cross' sufferer is like that. If this has happened to you, did you get a headache because you failed to get cross or was it because you got embarrassed in public and felt acutely enraged that your public image was dented? Work out in each case what you think it really was. Go over the incident with a friend if you're not sure or get together with a fellow headache sufferer and form a working team to check on each other's perceptions. Getting the right link is crucial. You could waste a lot of time acting out in the wrong way – getting cross when really you were embarrassed. When you are pretty sure what it was – and do try to be ruthless on yourself: if you don't the experiment won't work properly – go on to step three.

Step Three. Now, you have to test each hypothesis. First, though, have a look through your headache map and list of hypotheses. Some common patterns should strike you; if you find that you got an 'embarrassed → headache' chain only occasionally, and the 'failure to get cross → headache' chain very often, then this second one is the one to start with. Do you have any idea why you should be like this? Discuss it with your family or friends or doctor if you like – each person may give you some more clues to add to your developing picture – and then you can begin to change your behaviour.

The point is that whatever it is in your personal and neural system organisation that is causing your headache, it is going to be itself fairly well organised so that you have to break up this organisation and, in the process, integrate it with the rest of your functioning. Don't think about *not* being embarrassed in a kind of 'I will surmount it' sense, but think rather of the pattern that goes with it. Being embarrassed is quite a simple-sounding 'weakness' but ten-to-one there will be more behind it. To give you an insight into how to test hypotheses I will take an example of someone I know with the 'embarrassed' kind of problem and describe what she did.

Example:
The person involved was a 24-year-old secretary living at home with her divorced mother. Using the first two steps described above, she worked out that fear of being humiliated was causing most of her headaches and this is quite close to being 'embarrassed'. The first series of hypothesis tests went as follows:

   1. She decided to go into public areas – like supermarkets –

and deliberately put herself into humiliating situations and she felt it best if she had to do this for a whole week, every day. First off, she got a headache at the *thought* of doing it and called off the first three days of the week's test. Second, she found it impossible to *think* of humiliating situations for herself (now, for someone that sensitive and aware of humiliation, that was rich). So with her mother's help, she dreamt one up. She went to shop and deliberately left her purse at home (how humiliating!). Third, she again got a headache before buying anything and went home. Clues galore about how her headache functioned. Finally, she managed it and what did she find? Yes, she was acutely embarrassed, flushed. She arrived at the check-out counter with a big basket of things (having picked the meanest-looking cashier). As she pretended to search for her purse, she became angry, defensive and cynical. 'Well,' she snarled at last, looking at the cashier, 'you'll have to call the police – I've no money.' Expecting the worst, she glared round at everybody, and burst into tears. And what happened? Completely the reverse of what she had imagined.

'Everybody was terrific,' she reported later. 'The cashier was wonderful, she gave me a tissue, called the manager who insisted on driving me home himself to fetch my purse. In fact, everyone was so kind I daren't go in there again – I'd be too ashamed.'

2. She knew she had to do it again, though, at a different store in another part of town. And again, and again – until she could face one of her major problems in living: that her *fear* of people had been built up over the years in which she had imagined the worst. She was a fairly lonely person with few close friends and she resented other people and their lives. As a result she imagined they were sneering or laughing at her.

3. Once this particular hypothesis was broken open, it released a whole chain of secondary ones, all connected with her headache organisation. These had to be spelled out and tests for them devised. Included in this fresh set were:

i) She did not *look* at people properly. She kept her eyes down in public and her muscles tensed up immediately she felt a crowd of people's eyes on her. The strain of this seemed to bring on a headache.

ii) She never smiled at people – strangers, grocers etc – even if she saw them every day. She made no contact because she was shy.

iii) She never cried. She just felt bitter and angry with her lot in life. Actually, it wasn't so bad but she had never broken with her mother properly and spent too much time at home and often turned down dates because of this. Notice how the headache pattern was a symptom of far more than simple stress.

In each of the new areas she worked out tests of her own. For (i), for example, she made a point of watching people. Once she began to look properly at people, she discovered that few people *actually* looked at her and, if they did, it wasn't with hostility or cynicism. For (ii), she began to smile at people more and found that at first she was terrified of being talked to – 'I wouldn't know what to say' – and she was scared of drawing attention to herself. Being a brave girl, she forced herself to be more at ease with, and to learn to talk to, people better. Very quickly, she discovered that she *enjoyed* little informal chats rather than the long serious discussions she usually forced on people. Within a few months she had made friends at work with people who candidly told her later that earlier they'd thought she was very stuck-up and intellectual.

For (iii), she started accepting dates and found that she was very anxious about leaving her mother alone at night. They talked about it, had several fights, lots of upsets and tears and eventually became quite distant with each other. All of which upset the girl but she was compensated by the fact that she now had friends (including a boyfriend), had no headache and was engaging in facing problems in her life she had long avoided.

The point from this example is clear. Removing the headache was an emotionally costly process and certainly left the girl with a basketful of problems which took a long time to put right (if they ever will be). This is precisely how you know you have hit the right network: the girl was freed from a headache problem to attend to her living problems – her shyness, her lack of experience, depression, over-dependence on mother and gradual withdrawal from the world. By persevering with her investigation and realising slowly how complex the whole pattern was, she achieved a good result. This is how it usually works if you take the time and trouble and if you don't expect a quick trauma-free cure. Note, incidentally, that her 'cure' involved a whole range of inter-related actions; she had to examine her anxiety and relax; she had to *look* up at people (a physical response designed to inhibit the looking-down pose she inevitably adopted); she had to learn how to *be* with people and she had to learn how to cope with her family life.

We could go on with this particular case but there is no need. You can see how her pattern was slowly broken up as its complexity was unravelled and made sense of. By taking simple but nerve-wracking steps, she progressed to what I believe was a complete cure for headache. When I last saw her three years afterwards, she was happily married, living in another town and seeing her mother occasionally. Talk about twists of fate, though – her mother now suffers from headache.

You could ask, 'How could she be so hard on her mother?' and use that as an excuse for putting up with a bad situation. 'What about the mothers?' you may want to know, 'surely they count too?' A good point, because headache inevitably arises in situations which are full of emotion and involve other people whom you really feel you can't hurt or upset. Well, my feeling on this is clear. You have to decide: them or you. Their peace of mind or your headache. Sometimes it can mean a major upheaval and even unpleasant consequences, but sometimes (and in my experience, more often than not), *you* will push the other person into getting on and solving their own problems. More of this later.

Note how, in the example of the young woman that we used, a lot of things and levels were involved in the development of her headache and how much work had to be done to tap and change them all. This was a fairly complex example to use. Some headache complexes are quite a lot easier to disrupt. The important thing to remember is to go slowly and to at least start to explore your hypotheses even if it seems very tough to do at first. Once you get going, a whole lot of other things fall into line and the next steps follow on from them. Even if you don't hit the right hypothesis first time, it doesn't matter – there is usually enough information contained in them to lead you on to the right track for you. Try things on your own and if you get stuck, ask a friend to help – or your doctor. Basically, though, with perseverence and determination, there's no reason why you couldn't develop your own cure. In the next two chapters for more serious headache, there will be other clues and other examples to help and guide you along the way.

CHAPTER TWELVE

Towards a cure 2: Moderate-interference headache

Everything that was said in Chapter 11 applies to you but, given the nature of the way your headache interferes with your life, we have to go about things a bit differently. Most moderate sufferers have already developed their own hypotheses and chains of causes about their headaches and can quite easily talk about triggers and precipitating circumstances because they spend a lot of their time avoiding them. An added factor in their lives is that, by and large, they will have elicited a fairly large degree of secondary gain from their headache and be well-known at least in their families as 'headache' or 'migraine' people. Our way of seeking a cure here will therefore have to take into account these added factors.

The central point about 50-50 headache sufferers is that they seem to be like split people: capable of being perfectly normal and active one minute and then crippled the next by headache or migraine and all its misery. It is as if their lives are one long battle to break even and to resolve some deep, disturbing issue. One often feels like wishing they would either *be* normal all the time or have a chronic headache all the time. Then, at least, the struggle would be over.

Headaches for these people are the bane of their lives and if you think about this fact and the presence of a deep struggle within the personality of such people, two things strike you. First, having a headache so often means that the person is emotionally and sensorially deprived, since the time spent on headache is time wasted. Secondly, if you live like this you are only really being *half* a person. Now why? What, in this category, is the presence of the headache pattern telling us about the lives and personalities of the people who get them? If headache was a warning of problem areas in living for people in the mild category, what is being hinted at or suggested in the lives of moderate sufferers?

My conclusion is that while mild-frequency headache warns you about external problems that you must sort out, moderate frequency headache warns you about important aspects of your own biological functioning that must be attended to. Chronic headache or migraine – to take the argument further – is a warning that your biological functioning *as a whole* is in a state of disarray. If I'm correct in this, then basically the focus of attention for people in the moderate and chronic category is not so much your relationship with the outside world (although this is important) but should be more on yourself and on your relationships with people very close to you – your husband or wife, mother or father and children.

The difference between people in this category and the girl we used as an example in the last chapter is that she had the personal and biological capacity to live healthily. Her headaches were a way she had developed of registering frustration, fear and helplessness. Once these were removed, she got on with the job of *facing* her problems. She was well-equipped for the job, she just needed to arrange things to do it.

Moderate-frequency headache sufferers, by and large, not only have to arrange their lives to get on with the job but they also have to improve or learn the necessary skills to face up to problems. Having had headache or migraine for so long, having a partially deprived life has not given you enough time to learn how to function properly biologically. You are, in effect, partially 'frozen' inside. The trick is now to endeavour to give yourself that lost time so that lifting your headache can proceed apace while you make constructive use of your pain-free periods and your 50 per cent healthy part. For you, there really isn't going to be a 'quickie' cure and hard personal work and soul-searching is going to be an absolute must. So think

142

about it and once you've decided to take 'the cure', as it were, let's go. Grit your teeth – it helps to ease the pain.

Getting pain-free periods. The first thing you have to do is to have periods of pain-free time, quite substantial time, in fact, to work on yourself. To do that, you are going to need help. And help is available. Go and see your doctor and discuss with him ways and means of minimising the pain you suffer from headache. Note, not to minimise the frequency of your headache but to reduce the pain. You need the headache for investigative purposes but you certainly don't need the pain. If you have a satisfactory pain killer, no problem. If you don't, then discuss with your doctor which is likely to work. You may even like to consider one of the non-drug behavioural techniques to reduce the pain. Whatever you like – but do it. You might find that a tranquilliser or anti-depressant suits you best and they are fine. Use them under your doctor's guidance but just remember: you must be pain-free enough to think and not too drowsy or too drugged to stop thinking. Some anti-depressants like *amitriptyline* and some drugs with hypnotic effects, for example, are best taken at night so you sleep off the more extreme side-effects.

If you suffer from bouts of headache such as cluster head-ache or clusters of migraine attacks, you will have periods when you are headache-free. Don't waste those times – use them. Many people try to lead normal lives when they are headache-free, trying to forget about headache and to avoid them. In a way this is a pretence. If you get moderate-interference headache, even in cyclical bouts, it really is no good pretending that you're perfectly all right. You're not. And you basically need the time to explore yourself, so stop putting on the fronts.

Using your triggers properly. I'm going to assume that you have already established what triggers your headache. Some people *know* their triggers all right, but they have a love-hate relationship with them, avoiding them when they feel good and rebelling and indulging in them when they don't. I know one man who used to punish his wife at dinner parties by pretending to forget about his trigger and eating huge quantities of his *bête noir* food, knowing that they would have to leave early as a result. His wife loved going out but he didn't. I have met very few people in this category who don't know their triggers. So if you are the odd-man or woman out, sorry, go back a chapter and build up hypotheses and then come back.

Now, the thing with triggers is that *if* they are the real cause, then avoiding them should mean no headache, right? For the moment, leaving aside those triggers – like lights – which you can't avoid, how come your trigger works some times but not at others? If you have a clearly avoidable trigger, such as certain food, and if in avoiding it you get absolutely no headache, then obviously, you are allergic in some way to the food and your problems may be minimal.* But if it works some times and not others, then you have got to find out why. So here's what you do:

1. Think about your trigger: how you discovered it, how long it's been there, how reliable it is. Do you have doubts about it? Are there other things that might have a trigger function? Is there a whole series of related things that *might* be part of your pattern? Use your instincts again if you can, and probe the whole matter thoroughly. Did you find the trigger, or did someone tell you or did you read it somewhere? Many people jump to conclusions about their triggers without being absolutely certain and without testing them properly.

2. Assuming you're clear about your trigger or set of triggers, test them out to see if they really are causing your headache. First, write down the when, where and how of your last three attacks. Pay special attention to your state of mind *before* the attack and other precipitating conditions like *who* you were with, who you were going to see, and so on. Many triggers do not operate on their own but are really complex chains of events, one element of which you call the trigger. This is why sometimes they work and sometimes they don't. Key elements may sometimes be missing without your being aware of it; you

* I wouldn't like to say, however, that the matter closes for you here, if this is the case. No one yet knows the relationship between psychological and physical factors in such allergies or intolerances.

may have felt that you held or fought off a migraine when in fact, you didn't – you missed a stage. To help you test your triggers, here are two cases to illustrate the point.

Example 1

Michael J. believed his trigger was lying in bed on Sunday mornings. So to test it, he did two things. First, lucky chap, he took a week off work and lay in every morning – no migraine. Then he kept a record of other events that seemed relevant to his migraine and he did this for three months. Surprisingly enough, he noted that *if* his wife lay in with him, or *if* she was away (as she was on two Sundays, staying with her mother), he didn't get migraine. If, however, she was up and around, seeing to the family while he lay in bed, he got migraine. He checked on this over the next six months and found that lying in and hearing his wife about downstairs was really the trigger.

Try systematically exposing yourself to your trigger. Sometimes the act of knowing that you are deliberately testing yourself instead of avoiding a headache acts as a spurt and you don't get a headache. If this happens to you, calm down – you are not cured; you need a little more work. Here's another study:

Example 2

Maureen had a red wine migraine trigger. To test it, she went on her own to a wine bar and drank a glass. No headache. Delighted, she repeated the test with the same result, then went on a spree, convinced she was cured. For the next month she was fine. Then, at Christmas, she went out to a company dinner. With gay abandon, she ordered red wine and promptly got a migraine. Careful further investigation established that her trigger complex was (a) red wine, (b) a stuffy atmosphere, and (c) a high level of nervousness – she felt shy in the company of her bosses.

What about the unavoidable triggers like bright lights? Well, try this test. Go and hunt out bright lights at least once a day and *note* when you get a migraine. What I think happens with bright lights is that the pain of the light together with the visual disturbance only trigger migraine if you are feeling edgy or jumpy at the same time. Chronic migraine sufferers sense their edgy internal state and actually key themselves to be aware of bright lights. When one happens along, it completes a personal and nerve-system chain like a switch and sets you off. So, if you see bright lights when you're not edgy – no trigger. Likewise if you're edgy and see no bright lights. This leads conveniently on to a major concept I want to deal with.

Migraine or headache proneness. The point of the above discussion is to direct your attention to the fact that triggers are multi-complex. I believe that because of your personal and nerve-system handicaps, you carry around with you a type of functioning that is nearly always present quite independent to the act of getting a headache. Roughly put, you are prone to being edgy, anxious and tense, to watch other people and events for what they offer or give you in terms of prestige or security and to avoid situations that do not make you feel comfortable. You do not act on reality so much as react to it; your role in life is essentially passive. Whenever this fragile level of security or comfort is threatened, you get an increase in your general level of tension. When it gets too much, you'll get a headache and the obvious trigger you think causes your headache is usually the last straw, the last upsetting event. This is why so many fairly simple things appear to trigger headache and why the act of an ordinary bright light can sometimes push you over into a migraine attack and sometimes not. It's not the light alone, it's the final little bit of unfair, frustrating pain and its place in the sequence of events that pushes you over (or doesn't). If it comes early in a sequence, it will have a much lesser effect.

When I talk about using your trigger properly, what I mean is that you must try to build up the sequence accurately. In doing so you will automatically find yourself having to consider your own physical and emotional states and their relationship to external clues. The point of doing a trigger assessment is so that through it you can unearth that part of you or that

146

level of functioning which is nearly always there but which you have ignored through being concerned with avoiding headache attacks.

If you can learn to cope with the ebb and flow of your 'edgy' behaviour and know your trigger sequence accurately then there is a very good chance that you could cure your headache. Provided of course that you can *act* on the information properly; that is, with careful, systematic and slow application.

I won't pretend it's easy to switch from avoiding your triggers to using them as clues to find your 'edginess' but I do know that it is possible to do so. What is going to be the biggest hindrance is that you will not at first realise just how extensively edgy and insecure you are. Once you start mapping out your headaches and your preceding states of mind, you will literally hit an information mine, because just about everything will be a potential cause of upset. This may discourage you but if you want a cure, you'll have to go on because this is the real you your headaches have been warning you about. If you can't face it you will have to face perennial headache.

If my experiences are any guide, you should find disturbances in your functioning are essentially of a personal nature. Whatever the trigger, the underlying emotional and neural anxiety will have its roots in your day-to-day relationships. You might consider therefore mapping out how strong you feel (or how *boosted* as a person) day by day, and comparing that with both your edginess and your headache frequency. It can help you see the link. This is what one person found by doing this:

Example
This subject was a forty-five-year-old woman who tried mapping her 'high' feelings to see if they were linked to being headache-free. What she discovered, though, was a more complex picture. What made her feel 'strong' were comments and praise from people at work or casual acquaintances. By the time she went home, though, at the end of a day during which she had got a compliment, she had a severe tension headache.

147

By chance, however, her husband was called away one such day and she arrived home without knowing this and with a headache. Shortly after receiving the message, she noted that her headache had lifted. It was then that she realised something that she had known inside all along: her husband always reacted in a certain way to her excitement and good feeling at the praise she received. 'That's nice, dear,' he would say, completely disinterested. Then, later, he would always make some comment that pulled down her spirits. Her emotional security was too tied to her husband's approval and it was his *disapproval* that broke up a 'high' day. Further examination revealed a consistent relationship between her ups and downs with *him* and her headache.

Don't jump to the conclusion that *he* was the cause of her headache. It's not that simple. Her personality had been 'frozen' as I described in the chapter on migraine people and she related to everybody she came into contact with in a superficial way. Her level of central nervous system functioning was unstable and over-active. It was in a fairly constant state of flux, mixing anxiety and arousal as she constantly watched everybody for signs of approval or disapproval.* After a good day with 'highs', she felt so good, she actually relaxed because she felt 'safely confident'. In the state of ecstatic relaxation she was imminently vulnerable to disapproval, more so than

* How this works may be of interest to people with a similar pattern. How she coped with conflict and cohabitation (the need to behave with people and to feel safe) was by watching and processing the approval-disapproval data she received in a fixed and rigid manner. If she received negative data, she immediately spent all her mental energies trying to restabilise herself, either by justifying her actions (which had been criticised) or by finding fault with the person who criticised her. Favourable data were the 'highs' of the day, carefully stored, and the person giving them was constantly sought after. Fantasy images around and about that person would then preoccupy her time. It is these kinds of mental preoccupations that greatly reduce the headache sufferer's real mental abilities. If you fill your day with this kind of activity you'd end up as a mental wreck which is precisely the state you get into and that is what your headache is warning you about.

normal because her constant watching and reassuring herself was temporarily suspended. Under the stress of both the deep relaxation induced by the 'high' and suddenly or unexpectedly having to throw up her defence again (to face her husband) her system overloaded and headache followed. Her husband forced this conflict in her to happen more than anybody else did.

To ram home the point, let me say that I have often been able to find the same basic structure in people who have no husband or wife. One widowed woman I treated had exactly the same pattern in relation to her nine-year-old daughter. Other people have the same kind of complex relationship with aunts, uncles, mothers, fathers, children, bosses, the lot.

I will concede that some people won't easily be able to get to the point where their triggers have been explored properly. Quite apart from the fact that you'll need help to keep going, some of the finer points of analysis may be too upsetting and overwhelming. You might find that going to see your doctor and/or a psychotherapist who works either with headache people or with problems in general, a great help in getting through the emotions and difficulties involved. Whatever the limitations of psychotherapy, it definitely has its place in the treatment of headache and this, I believe, is it. Try to find someone who is kind and understanding *and* pushy. The sympathy bit is all very nice and comforting at first, but remember you have a job to do and you need someone who is going to keep your nose to the grindstone while you find your own cure. Sometimes, behavioural scientists attached to university psychology or psychiatry departments are only too willing to help you find your triggers and to map your headaches. So ask your doctor if you're interested.

Going on the offensive
Now what? We'll assume everything's proceeded quite well so far and that it's time now for the change over. Where do you begin? Mainly, it depends on you and the fragility of your personal environment. It's best to start with the easiest thing to

do and let the effects gradually spread. I think you'll have to concern yourself with:

1. A combination of over-excitation and under-excitation of your nervous system. You will get too active and swing to being too 'at ease' without having stages in between – you'll be either flat-out or dead-slow. This will mean that:

2. You won't relax properly overall. This does *not* mean that you can't sleep or laze around. I find many moderate interference and chronic headache sufferers are past-masters at creative laziness. They seem to be active or busy while really loafing around, day-dreaming and so on. Proper relaxation does not mean flopping out or tensing and relaxing the muscles of your body – as, for example, the relaxation therapists teach you – this is a simple relaxation. Proper system relaxation means that you give your body's psychosomatic *organisation* a rest, *not* simply by sleeping, but by changing the organisation, using components in different orders or sequences, doing something completely different and, more importantly, in a different way. To relax means to take your mind off the usual run of things, to let your mind rest through *change*. What is the usual run of things for the headache sufferer? Watching, defending, being edgy, tense, competitive and so on. So what would be a *rest* from these things? Correct: to stop watching, being defensive, being edgy and so on. Too many people think resting from their jobs or the children is what matters. It isn't. You must relax and rest away from your own 'bad' habits.

I often ask headache sufferers how they relax and the answer they give is: 'play golf, chess or take evening classes, join women's groups', etc, etc. Examination reveals that these things are just as bad as their jobs. They bring the same old hack headache organisation to bear with the same old inevitable results. To back up my argument, let me just mention that sleep researchers have discovered that migraine sufferers don't sleep the same way as other people do.

There are two basic sleep stages – deep sleep in which your mind really takes a break, and rapid eye movement (REM) sleep in which your mind is partially awake. In this second

150

phase, you go over the events of the day, think about things and so on. It's adaptive, active sleep and probably accounts for the way you can go to sleep with a problem and wake up with a solution. Like a computer, your mind continues to function – often better because it is unhampered by your anxiety and other emotional interferences. Headache sufferers tend to have more of this REM sleep (Dexter & Weitzman, 1970; McGrath and Cohen, 1978) than normal, which can make you feel pretty dynamic, huh? Until you're told that (a) you have too much REM sleep, and (b) you need the deep sleep as much as the REM sleep. Headache sufferers, it is clear, actually do the same thing in their *sleep* as they do when they're awake. Is there no stopping them?

3. You won't really know either yourself or people properly. You will live on the surface and, to change things, you will have to get to know yourself better. And your spouse, and your friends. You will have to become more sensitive. *Sensitive*, by the way – not easily upset.

4. You probably ignore a large number of running problems and glaring inconsistencies in your life; anxieties and fears that overwhelm you from time to time quite separate from your headache. You probably bemoan your fate a lot, worry about the world and make yourself sometimes very depressed indeed.

That's enough troubles to begin with. Now to put them together with your triggers and develop treatment programmes.

Treatment

Now, I don't know which area you are going to be able to work on best. Some people have wonderful partners who *really* want to help and who take an active part in the proceedings, even if it means they have to change as well. Others get no help at all from their partners. This is something you'll have to decide yourself. What I'm going to do here is to spell out what you have to do and give you some suggestions in each area. Remember, even if you start in one area, you must gradually try to involve all the areas we have mentioned. The 'cure' depends on your acting and changing in a complex, multi-level way. I'll also tell you as we go which of the therapeutic techniques available might help you achieve your goal.

Stabilising your level of central nervous system functioning. What would you do if you had to stop looking and watching people? Never thought about it? Now's the time. Try this set of exercises on a quiet day when you haven't got a headache:

1. Imagine that everyone you met did to you what you do to them. How would you feel?

2. Imagine what would happen if all the people that frightened you died. Relieved? *Don't* feel guilty – it's just a game.

3. Look at everyone in your office or on your bus or train. Imagine tickling the most serious-looking people.

Ridiculous? Maybe, but note what happened to your state of mind: it lightened momentarily. You don't play with images and moods and ideas enough; you don't have proper fantasies and wishes; you don't have fun. If you're going to calm your bodily functioning down you will have to replace the constant alertness you live with by some other mental activity, both to balance your long-established state of alertness and to begin to inhibit it. You need to expand your imagination, to follow impulses and ideas more in order to break up your obsession with your watching. Systematic desensitisation – remember it? we discussed it earlier – might well help you here to do this and it is worth going into.

Here's a list of alternate obsessions which can be used to break your pathological one. Don't be put off by the word 'obsession'. Getting obsessed with a different thing is sometimes the only way to counterbalance the original one. The trick is to keep shifting your obsessions so they don't get entrenched:

1. Some people find getting obsessed with their personal appearance helps to break the old chain.

2. Getting obsessed with sexual matters works for a great many people. Plan an affair if you like (in fantasy only – the reality could be disastrous), examine your friends' sex lives (in your head). Both are things almost always guaranteed to

152

intrigue you and to break your preoccupation with security.

3. Be actively lazy. Why not? You are capable of that, surely? Worried what people will think? Then be cunningly lazy.

4. Don't talk so much. Try proper listening. Many headache sufferers talk too much and seldom listen to what other people say.

Relaxation therapy may be of use in slowing your general level of arousal down. If you combined it with trying to develop new obsessions and new thought processes, you could do yourself a lot of good. However, remember the whole point is to reduce both extremes of your functioning, to build in stages and steps on the way. If you're going to stop being over-excited or over-watchful, you've also got to stop being under-excited. How do you do this? You review and re-examine your relaxation outlets and how you take things easy. This is best discussed under the next heading.

Re-structuring your activity levels. At the simplest level, you could proceed by ensuring that you're getting a good night's sleep. Personally, I think this has been a very neglected part of headache treatment so let's correct that right away. There are several possible ways of doing this. Control your sleep time so that you get to bed tired. Don't lie in – it tends to break up patterns – and don't sleep during the day. Best, though, is to look up the nearest sleep research laboratory to you and volunteer for assessment. That way, you'll find out if you're over-doing REM sleep and there are drugs you can take to correct this. You can also be trained to increase your deep sleep capability. If you don't want to go to these lengths, just see your doctor and discuss it with him.

Next, examine your sports, hobbies and interests. You should play at least one *team* game a week. And not, please, croquet. Volley-ball is great for headache sufferers because it is too fast for careful thought, requires instinct, physical awareness and co-ordination *and* involves intimate physical and psychological actions. All of these are usually underdeveloped in headache sufferers. Of course, if you really want to, try all-in wrestling:

153

they tell me it's a very interesting sport. Avoid golf, jogging, cricket, tennis and the like, to begin with – they are too slow, isolated and demand the wrong organisation of skills. Football is okay, but stay out of goal. Don't play anything on a serious basis. Stay with the strugglers, the reserves and the like.

Hobbies. Well, disco-dancing, believe it or not, is 'cool' for headache sufferers for similar reasons as volley-ball. Same goes for being an active football *fan*. All that yelling and screaming out in the cold is good for you. Your hobbies should be active, involving you in movement and, preferably, change too. If you are an accountant or any other such staid 'establishment' figure, you need a complete change. Try dancing in a chorus line, singing in the local pub or acting. Anything that taxes you, frightens you or stimulates you in different ways. If you're a disc jockey with a headache problem, try something completely different like mountain climbing or canoeing. You could also try taking a job as a part-time librarian. The change of pace could upset you creatively and help you stop being 'on the outside, looking in' – to coin one of your phrases.

You also need relaxations at different levels. Don't use every spare moment in doing your hobby, sleeping or watching television, doing your charity bit and interspersing them with sneaked periods of laziness. Develop your laziness. Stop hiding it for a start and *be* self-obsessed – for you, not for others. Go and sit on a beach or in the park and deliberately do nothing. Rebel against the little voice inside that keeps saying, 'You're *wasting* time.' Part of the headache sufferers' psychological appreciation of his or her failure to relax in proper stages is that everything, in order for it to be allowed, has to have a purpose. So many headache sufferers do things because they feel it will 'benefit' them, make them more interesting, healthy, etc, when in fact a lot of the time the activities make them more *boring*. You have to start doing irrelevant things, flippant things, things that cause people to look down their noses at you. Here are some irrelevant 'hobbies' to get you started:

1. Look vacuously into space at dinner parties.
2. Be actively boring to selected people. That is great fun.

3. Cultivate a refined ignorance.

4. Try your hand at different roles. Be breezy and irrelevant one day, then loud, then shy, then weak, then aggressive. You may puzzle people close to you – practise on strangers first – but you will open up a lot of insights and feelings about yourself.

5. Yawn a lot.

6. Go back to chapter 11 and look at the list of expressive outlets (giggling, etc) and work your way through them.

7. Carry a comic around with you. Or movie magazine. If you're not that brave, carry a comic *and* Tolstoy. Be prepared to defend your reading matter with copious argument.

Enough. You may have noticed that while each is irrelevant, each gently makes *fun* of *you* and tests and stretches your ability to *relax* your obsessions with watching how people see you. If you can't do them, you'll have to find out why. Don't take yourself and life so seriously. You must learn to play in the fullest sense of the word and to relax your embedded organisation.

Improving your relationships and attending to real problems. My guess is that most people with severe headaches divide their relationships into two: their close relationships versus their relationships with the rest of the world. You watch the rest of the world obsessively and you take for granted your home life. You try to keep everyone at home as quiet and ordered and routine as possible, freeing you to worry about the outside world. What you should be doing is keeping the outsiders quiet and stable while worrying and attending to the inside world at home – that is, yourself, your relationships with your spouse, your children, family and friends. The real meat of living – and by that I mean *problem facing* – is in your relationships to those closest to you. And do you know why? What can *you* do to change the world – even the world of your office or the bus queue? *Answer:* nothing. So why worry about the outside world's problems or even what the world is coming to? Where you can be really effective and change things is in facing the problems that come up in your personal relations. So it stands to reason that *this* is where you should start to focus your interests.

I would like to go on and spell out some suggestions about how to proceed in this area but it really is too big a topic to treat properly in a book of this size. Psychotherapy, counselling, even marriage guidance can help you to look at yourself properly and at your marriage. And of course, you can do it on your own by thinking and testing out ideas. In the next chapter, too, we'll touch on this subject briefly. What I will do, though, in closing, is to detail some of the problem areas you must concern yourself with along the way. Mind how you go though! Some of the problems are very delicate:

1. How do you get *angry*? How does your husband or wife get angry? If you *don't* ever get angry, I say HAH! Have a close look at the ways you cope with anger and frustration and you'll soon discover hundreds of devious little tricks you use to express it. Do you break things? Are you accident-prone or clumsy? Do you confuse anger with fear? Do you know how to get really, flaming mad? If you don't – find out why.

2. Do you hate *extreme* displays of emotion? Why? Are you affectionate? Are you sexually affectionate? Do you know the difference between the two? What about your partner? There are many good books on these issues that *really* open your eyes. *Tip for men* – start reading all the women's magazines you can lay your hands on. No, not *girly* magazines, *their* (women's) magazines. Just about every issue of the 'glossies' contain pages of advice, articles *and* extracts from current books written by top psychologists and psychiatrists. Find out what books are available. Read them.

3. Do you enjoy things with those closest to you? Do you enjoy watching your children grow up and experience all the trials and tribulations of living, or do you smother them? Do you share your fantasies and ideas (sexual or otherwise) with your partner or do you keep them to yourself? Do you use your children or your partner to avoid developments or changes that you should be engaging in? Think about all these things.

In trying to touch on each area, I have focused on what I

have found to be the most important issues involved. I could be wrong or what I have had to say may not specifically work for you. Don't haggle too much with this, though, because what I really want to get across is the *kind* of things that you will have to do to shift that headache or migraine organisation. Try out your own ideas; work with a doctor or therapist; do whatever will work for you. Remember, the operative word is to *organise* your activity better. I would love to hear about what *you* did that worked, even if it is the opposite of what I have said. It really is more important to test and explore than to be *right*.

CHAPTER THIRTEEN

Towards a cure 3: Major or chronic interference headache

I haven't got a great deal to say about people in this category, not for lack of ideas of theories or practical advice, but because people with chronic headache really do need a lot of work under quite close supervision of a trained professional. I have yet to come across a chronic sufferer who has, by their own efforts, 'cured' their headache. What I think must be said, however, is a word or two about the directions a possible cure should take and what I have found to be the key problems involved in their treatment. We need to know *what* we are dealing with very clearly because misconceptions at the basic level of understanding have created, in the past, much of the confusion that exists about headache and its preventative treatment.

First we must accept that major-interference headache, be it muscle-contraction or migraine-based, is a pathological condition not to be dismissed lightly simply because it does little *physical* damage to the organism. By definition, if the major-interference pattern is long-standing, and especially if it began in adolescence, you have a person who has not developed full adult physical and psychological patterns of dealing with cohabitation and conflict. Having a disruptive headache pattern *means* that one's life is disrupted. You can't grow, think, act or develop properly. You are handicapped. I hope that if this book has done nothing else, it has helped readers to appreciate how pervasive and thorough-going headache effects are on the biological organism in direct proportion to the pattern of disruption. The more frequent and interfering the headache, the tighter the organisation and the more widespread the accompanying psychosomatic pathology. We must start accepting that, in chronic cases, *mental* damage is one consequence of this.

Secondly, we are dealing with something systematic, not a minor trauma or infection. The sufferer's personal and neural system functioning is organised badly. We must seek its manifestation in the whole current functioning of the individual and look for its roots in the sufferer's characteristic *learned* ways of dealing with reality. To 'cure' the condition, we must first control the symptoms then establish the extent of the problem and finally proceed to teaching the sufferer a better organisation and better ways of dealing with reality. Headache people successfully learned their headache organisation – it can also be successfully unlearned. But only if we are all (sufferers and doctors) prepared to come to terms with the complexity of headache. A complex problem requires complex, tough and thorough-going solutions and we must, all of us, be prepared to work hard, explore and research, take risks even, to get there.

Stages in the cure theory
Prophylactic drugs. Without pain reduction or headache-free periods, nobody can work at their headache. Drug research is pushing along nicely and the new thinking in pain will have its inevitable benefits in the future (Merskey, 1976). What I think needs attention, though, and where, with careful work, breakthroughs for helping headache sufferers (note: helping, not curing) may be closer than we realise, is in the development of drugs to aid sleep. Let me explain. Quite apart from the sleep disturbances detailed in the last chapter that headache sufferers experience, sleep is an efficient but temporary cure on its own. Children with headache or migraine automatically fall asleep to stop attacks. Once patterns develop, they, like adults, seek sleep-like relief. They lie down spontaneously (without any parental instruction) in darkened

159

rooms and try to sleep. This, together with avoiding bright light and noise, etc, are attempts to cut down on the person's sensory input and activity level. One can argue that they arise out of attempts to minimise pain or nausea, which I think is partially true, but it seems to me more likely that they are all part of an attempt-to-sleep pattern which is well-established in children but disrupted in adults. Children sleep spontaneously as a reaction to stress or trauma. Adults *should* do the same but *autonomic* functioning in adults is tightly bound to social and cultural contexts, not to spontaneous rhythms. It follows therefore that sleep is a natural restorative whose benefits should be explored, not only in the preventative sense of helping chronic sufferers achieve nightly deep sleep (as opposed to over-active REM sleep) but also in the symptom-relieving sense of helping those prepared or able to take sleep time both to use it on its own and to facilitate the action of any analgesic taken.

Prophylactic relearning. Sleep helps organisational learning. When you sleep, you replay the trauma in a more natural, fantasy-like and play-like way. Children's lives have the same quality – reality is muted and blended with fantasy so that new adjustments can be practised or tried out in safe, playful contexts. Healthy adults should have carried this learning pattern through so that their sleep, their reflective and relaxation adult patterns contain significant components of the child's, reintegrated and redefined to suit the demands of reality. Severe headache sufferers are disturbed in all these functions. It follows, therefore, that the major treatment offensive must be to re-establish the adult sufferer's ability to do these things.

What happens to a child who gets upset or frightened and who can't regress into a reflective, playful, safe haven – either in him or herself, or in his or her relationship to a parent? Over time, they do two things: one, they develop suitable stress signs like headache as I described in Chapter 8; two, they try to stop their world from frightening them. A child who can perform healthy regressions doesn't *bend* his or her reality to cope. They don't have to. They have a safe, fantasy-play haven,

160

so reality therefore becomes the shaper or arbiter of their development. Severe headache sufferers have carried through into adult life the reality-avoidance pattern we see in child sufferers and made of *it*, a life-style.

Headache sufferers shut down or diminish their sensory and emotional input to a level that doesn't frighten them. Thus they need to be taught how to achieve normal regression play-fantasy levels *and then* to expand their sensory and emotional input so that they can learn to react to fear properly without using their headache organisation. They must finally learn to put the two together: reality contact, and a proper regressive organisation. When something upsets you – cry. When you're angry – *be* angry. When sad, *be* sad, etc, etc. It sounds simple, but, believe me, headache people haven't learnt the steps on the way so they don't know how or when to cry, to get angry and so on. To know *when*, you have to attend to broad sensory input (to *see* what is upsetting you) and to know *how* you have to attend to your reactions (to be able to get upset properly and appropriately).

The fact that headache sufferers have too much REM sleep is very significant. As I understand it, it is a valuable clue (sometimes the only one) to what they are struggling to do inside. They have over-activity in sleep because in waking they do not try out and explore and experiment enough with the world. The REM sleep is an indicator that their body *needs* to explore, play, etc, and in sleeping, the central nervous systems of these people try to make up for the conscious deficit. Improve a sufferer's conscious activities in the correct way and the REM sleep level goes down to normal.

All that I have written in the preceding two chapters is based on this formulation, and mild to moderate sufferers are, I think, able to take the steps I have outlined, which, among other things, create the right learning. However, chronic or severe sufferers have to start virtually from scratch. Moderate sufferers have a partially healthy organisation which needs to be mobilised for treatment. But chronics have no healthy organisation; it has to be taught. What follows is a rough outline of how this might be done, given that prophylactic or symptomatic behavioural interventions have already been used to create pain-free periods.

We are dealing with a problem that has become obscured, both for the person and for those who suffer with him or her, by the secondary, psychological and social gains or reactions to the headache experience. Any cure will have to slice through these layers of sympathy, passive-aggression, hostility, over-dependency, fear and so on to get at the real problem. So I envisage some kind of psychosocial surgery to peel away the secondary effects. I won't trouble with this here because, firstly, it alone is a major job and one that requires very careful psychotherapy and management. Secondly, strangely, it might not be a necessary component of 'cure'. Frankly, a person's ability to get through this kind of intervention determines their 'curability'. All too many people have, by their thirtieth birth-day, embedded themselves in comfy, headache-making re-lationships that are often impossible to shift. Even if they are willing, often their partners are not. Far better, I believe, to start with the basic bodily re-training and try to tie in gains made there with the person's personal relationships. I have occasionally achieved a partial 'cure' by encouraging the suf-ferer to lead a 'second life' alongside their home life, to make new friends who are able to tolerate their new skills and, more important, new forms of emotional expression (Lambley, 1976).

Structured relaxation training, assertive training, systematic desensitisation are all steps in the right direction to help the person learn a new organisation. But as they stand at the moment, they are too general and too unrelated to what actually happens in the way headache sufferers think and behave. We need much finer and more individual re-training programmes to get at the deficits involved. Let me spell out, therefore, one or two of the techniques I have used or am in the process of developing:

1. Chronic headache sufferers are often physically poorly co-ordinated. They can't play games, as I advised in the last

chapter, and so miss out all the learning benefits to be had there. They can, however, be trained from scratch. I often used to take a large ball and toss it to my headache patients so that they could see how poor their dexterity and co-ordination is. Making them practise every day until they improved and ignoring their complaints, their hostility ('Really, does it *matter* if I can't reach a ball?') and their attempts to àvoid the task ('Really, who has time for something as *mindless* as ball-throwing?') is one step on the way to opening out their ability to make better physical contact with the world. You won't believe how many headache sufferers are literally *terrified* of things the rest of us face day-in and day-out. Going for a walk, going out alone, going to the shop, are sometimes very debilitating experiences. Once they get started, though, they get obsessed and delighted in a child-like way with how *silly* they've been. All of which can be used to build on if other people can show them how nice it is to do and how nice it is to admit to being *silly*.

2. Free a chronic sufferer from responsibility and stress for two weeks, either by having them to stay (not so good) or by arranging a 'special' holiday and interesting things begin to happen. For one, they sleep more, laze around more and actually begin to seek out feared situations to see how they'd cope. All of which can be built on and structured accordingly for when they go back home.

3. When things first upset or frighten you, you tend to be quite extreme in your reactions. You panic, over-react and so on. What often happens to people who develop problems in living is that their first over-reactions of fear are themselves over-reacted to by people in their environment. If I get a fright and scream and you were frightened by my scream and you scream louder than me – even though you haven't yet seen what frightened me – it would be very easy for both of us to get lost in calming *you* down rather than me. This is very like what happens to headache sufferers and they have to be re-educated and shown how to cope with their *own* fears rather than attending to others. As a preliminary measure, I have found it

possible to train headache sufferers to obsessively fixate on their own distress by de-sensitising them to criticism, social disapproval and by literally teaching them how to cry, get angry and so on and by allowing them the time alone to do so without fear of consequences. In some cases, it is possible to reverse the sufferer's own learned social pattern by teaching the people in his or her environment to refuse to attend to any headache symptom and only to attend to any other sign of regressive stress, like rage, crying and so on. I have found this technique very effective in adolescents or older children where parents provide very influential feedback for the child. In some cases, however, husbands or wives can be instructed to do the same.

Don't think these techniques work on their own. In the last example, for instance, teaching a person to cry properly or to express proper emotions is only one stage. Each new gain has to be built on the one before and everything tied together to create the necessary impact on the headache organisation. Every level has to be applied and blended with the next one according to a sequence and pattern defined by the individual and his or her environment. Remember, the more severe the headache interference, the more levels have to be used in treating it and the more extensive the research needed to find and operate them.

Last, last word

This has been a brief but, I hope, practical look at the current state of the headache field. I have tried to provide a fair cross-section of the major developments in thinking and to cover the most important treatment modes available. It is an interesting area to work in because, by and large, once adequately informed of where they stand, headache sufferers are a dogged and determined lot and more than other patients can be relied upon to get on with the job. I hope this book helps you to do that, if only in a small way.

Brief Glossary

Arteries

The blood vessels that carry blood away from the heart to the extremities of the body. Arterial: pertaining to arteries. Arterial disease: disease in the blood vessels.

Autonomic nervous system

The part of the nervous system responsible for arousing the various organs and systems of the body and for relaxing them. The autonomic nervous system regulates the body's general level of functioning.

Blood vessels

These are either arteries or veins and are the pipe-like things that carry blood around the body.

Brain scanners

These are machines which make maps of the various areas of the brain. Their technical name is Computerised Axial Tomographs.

Central nervous system

This refers to the entire bodily network of nerves and their connections.

Cerebral

Refers to the brain. Cerebral cortex: the major part of the brain.

Cerebrospinal fluid

The fluid that holds the brain in place and acts as a cushion to protect it and the nerves in the spinal column.

Cohabitation

The task of living together in peace and community.

Conflict management

The task of managing disputes and arguments.

165

Conversional state

This refers to the mental state when a person 'converts' a mental anxiety into an apparently physical symptom.

Delusional state

This is the state in which a person believes things in the real world to be different to what they actually are. This is in contrast to the hallucinatory state in which the person believes things to be real which are not actually there.

Dizygotic

Refers to twins coming from the same ovum but different eggs.

Gastro-intestinal

Referring to the stomach and the intestinal regions.

Genetic

Refers to the process of inheritance.

Hypochondriacal state

This is when a person believes he or she is suffering from an illness when they are not.

Lesion

The term used to describe a change in the state of an area in the body. It can refer to a tumour, an abscess, or other injury.

Monozygotic

Refers to twins coming from the same egg.

Nausea

The state of feeling sick, as opposed to vomiting, the act of being sick.

Neural

Of or relating to nerves and the nervous system.

Para-sympathetic nervous system

This is the part of the autonomic nervous system concerned with relaxing the body's various components.

Prophylactic

This refers to treatment that aims at preventing the occurrence of illness. It is in contrast to symptomatic treatment that deals with specific symptoms.

Somatic

Bodily functions, pertaining to the body.

Structure

A word that here is used to refer to the way components of various entities are put together or organised.

Sympathetic nervous system

This is the part of the autonomic nervous system that deals with co-ordinating the arousal of the body's various components.

Vascular

Of or relating to blood vessels.

Vasoconstriction

This is narrowing of the blood vessels. Vasconstrictors are drugs which produce this effect.

Vasodilation

This is the swelling of the blood vessels.

Veins

These are the blood vessels that take blood from the various organs of the body and return it to the heart by way of the lungs.

References

Bakal, D. A. 'Headache: A biopsychological perspective'. *Psychological Bulletin*, 1975, 82, 369–382.

Bickerstaff, E. R. 'Basilar artery migraine'. *Lancet*, 1961, 1, 15.

Bille, B. 'Headache in children'. In P. J. Vinken & G. W. Bruyn (Eds.) *Handbook of Clinical Neurology. Volume 5*, Amsterdam: North Holland, 1968.

Blackwell, B. 'Hypertensive crisis due to monoamineoxidase inhibitors'. *Lancet*, 1963, 2, 849–850.

Cocklin, C. 'Migraine'. *British Medical Journal*, 1978, November.

Crane, G. 'Clinical pharmacology in its twentieth year'. In R. Cancro (Ed.) *The Schizophrenia Syndrome*, New York: Brunner Mazel, 1975.

Curran, D. A., Hinterberger, H., & Lance, J. W. 'Methysergide'. In A. P. Friedman (Ed.) *Research and Clinical Studies in Headache. Volume I*, Basel: Karger, 1967.

Dengrove, E. 'Behavior therapy of headache'. *American Journal of Psychosomatic Dentistry and Medicine*, 1968, 15, 14–18.

Dexter, J. D., & Weitzmann, E. D. 'The relation of nocturnal headaches to sleep stage patterns'. *Neurology*, 1970, 20, 513–518.

Ehyia, A., & Fenichel, G. M. 'The natural history of acute confusional migraine'. *Archives of Neurology*, 1978, 35, 368–369.

Fine, B. D. 'Psychoanalytic aspects of headpain'. In A. P. Friedman (Ed.) *Research and Clinical Studies in Headache. Volume 2*, Basel: Karger, 1969.

Friar, L. R., & Beatty, J. 'Migraine: Management by trained

control of vasoconstriction'. *Journal of Consulting and Clinical Psychology*, 1976, 44, 46–53.

Friedman, A. P. 'Headache'. In A. M. Friedman & H. I. Kaplan (Eds.) *Comprehensive Textbook of Psychiatry*. Baltimore: Williams and Wilkins, 1975.

Gainotti, G., Cianchetti, C., & Taramelli, M. 'Anxiety level and psychodynamic mechanisms in medical headaches'. In A. P. Friedman (Ed.) *Research and Clinical Studies in Headache. Volume 3*, Basel: Karger, 1972.

Green, J. E. 'A survey of migraine in England'. *The Migraine Trust*, London, 1975.

Hungerford, G. D., Du Boulay, G. H., & Zilkha, K. J. 'Computerised axial tomography in patients with severe migraine'. *Journal of Neurology, Neurosurgery and Psychiatry*, 1976, 39, 990–994.

Klein, D. F., & Davis, J. M. *Diagnosis and Drug Treatment of Psychiatric Disorders*, Baltimore: Williams and Wilkins, 1969.

Klimek, A., Szulc-Kuberska, J., & Kawiorski, S. 'Lithium therapy in cluster headaches'. *European Neurology*, 1979, 18, 267–268.

Knight, G. 'Surgical treatment of migraine'. In P. J. Vinken & G. W. Bruyn (Eds.) *Handbook of Clinical Neurology. Volume 5*, Amsterdam: North Holland, 1968.

Lambley, P. 'The use of assertive training and psychodynamic insight in the treatment of migraine headache'. *Journal of Nervous and Mental Disease*, 1976, 163, 61–64.

Lance, J. W. *Headache*, London: Butterworth, 1978.

Mathews, W. B. *Practical Neurology*, Oxford: Blackwell, 1970.

McGrath, M. J., & Cohen, D. B. 'REM sleep facilitation of adaptive waking behaviour: A review of the literature'. *Psychological Bulletin*, 1978, 85, 24–57.

Mersky, H. 'The status of pain'. In O. W. Hill (Ed.) *Modern Trends in Psychosomatic Medicine. Volume 3*, London: Butterworths, 1976.

Miller, N. 'Learning of visceral and glandular responses'. *Science*, 1969, 163, 434–445.

Mitchell, K. R., & Mitchell, D. M. 'Migraine: An exploratory treatment application of programmed behaviour therapy techniques.' *Journal of Psychosomatic Research*, 1971, 15, 137–157.

Neligan, P., Harriman, D. G. F., & Pearce, J. 'Respiratory arrest in familial hemiplegic migraine: A clinical and neuropathological study'. *British Medical Journal*, 1977, September, 732–734.

Ogden, H. D. 'Headache studies; statistical data'. *Journal of Allergy*, 1952, 23, 58.

Paulley, J. W., & Haskell, D. A. L. 'The treatment of migraine without drugs'. *Journal of Psychosomatic Research*, 1975, 19, 367–374.

Pearce, J. *Modern Topics in Migraine*, London: Heinemann, 1975.

Petersen, J., Scruton, D., & Dounie, A. W. 'Basilar artery migraine with transient atrial fibrillation'. *British Medical Journal*, 1977, October, 1125–1126.

Prensky, A. L., & Sommer, D. 'Diagnosis and treatment of migraine in children.' *Neurology*, 1979, 29, 506–510.

Rawson, M. D., & Liversedge, L. A. 'The clinical pharmacology of migraine'. In J. Pearce (Ed.) *Modern Topics in Migraine*, London: Heinemann, 1975.

Refsum, S. 'Genetic aspects of migraine'. In P. J. Vinken & G. W. Bruyn (Eds.) *Handbook of Clinical Neurology. Volume 5*, Amsterdam: North Holland, 1968.

Sargent, J. D., Green, E. E., & Walters, E. D. 'The use of autogenic feedback in a pilot study of migraine and tension headaches'. *Headache*, 1972, 12, 120–124.

Simons, W. 'Symptoms and suicide'. *Psychiatric. Quarterly*, 1969, January, 327–329.

Somerville, B. W. 'A study of migraine in pregnancy'. *Neurology* (Minneapolis), 1972, 22, 824.

Thrush, D. 'Treatment of migraine'. *British Medical Journal*, 1978, October, 1004–1005.

Waters, W. E. 'Epidemiology of migraine'. In J. Pearce (Ed.) *Modern Topics in Migraine*, London: Heinemann, 1975.

Wolff, H. G. *Headache and Other Head Pain*, London: Oxford University Press, 1972.

Wolpe, J. *Psychotherapy by Reciprocal Inhibition*, Johannesburg: University of the Witwatersrand Press, 1958.

Interesting other work on headache and related topics

Nobody, I think, should be put off by technical or medical-sounding articles or books. The references overleaf are the major ones available now and you should approach them armed with a good, popular medical or psychological dictionary (a good one to buy is *Pears Medical Encyclopaedia* by J. A. C. Brown, London: Sphere Books, 1977). The same goes for the books in the following list:

Beatty, E. T., & Haynes, S. N. 'Behaviour intervention with muscle-contraction headache: A review'. *Psychosomatic Medicine*, 1979, 41, 165–180.

Cohen, D. B. *Sleep and Dreaming*, Oxford: Pergamon, 1979.

Cohen, M. J. *et al* 'Evidence for response stereotypy in migraine headache'. *Psychosomatic Medicine*, 1978, 40, 344–354.

Diamond, S. 'Depressive headaches'. *Headache*, 1964, 4, 255.

Diamond, S. *et al, Vasoactive Substances Relevant to Migraine*, Springfield: C. C. Thomas, 1975.

Diamond, S., & Furlong, W. B. *More Than Two Aspirin*, Chicago: Follet, 1976.

Evans, P. *Mastering your Migraine*, London: Granada, 1978.

Freese, P. *Headaches, The Kinds And The Cures*, London: Allen and Unwin, 1976.

Grenell, R. G., & Gabay, S. *Biological Foundations of Psychiatry*, New York: Raven Press, 1976.

Hanington, E. *Migraine*, London: Priory, 1974.

Hartman, E. L. *The Function of Sleep*, New Haven: Yale University Press, 1973.

Hill, O. W. *Modern Trends in Psychosomatic Medicine*, London: Butterworths, 1976.

Lipowski, Z. J. 'Psychosomatic medicine in the seventies: an overview'. *American Journal of Psychiatry*, 1977, 134, 233–244.

Medina, J. L., & Diamond, S. 'The clinical link between migraine and cluster headaches'. *Archives of Neurology*, 1977, 34, 470–472.

McQuade, W., & Aikman, A. *How to Stop Your Mind Killing Your Body*, London: Hutchinson, 1976.

Migraine: Mystery and Misery, London: The Migraine Trust, 1975.

Price, K. P. 'The application of behaviour therapy to the treatment of psychosomatic disorders'. *Psychotherapy*, 1974, 11, 138–155.

Rees, W. L. 'Personality and psychodynamic mechanisms in migraine'. *Psychotherapy and Psychosomatics*, 1974, 23, 111–122.

Sachs, O. W. *Migraine*, New York: University of California Press, 1970.

Schwartz, G. E., & Weiss, S. M. 'What is behavioural medicine?' *Psychosomatic Medicine*, 1977, 39, 377–381.

Sherwin, D. 'A new method for treating "headache" '. *American Journal of Psychiatry*, 1979, 136, 1181–1183.

Sternbach, R. A. *Pain: A Psychophysiological Analysis*. New York: Academic Press, 1968.

Warnes, H. 'An integrative model for the treatment of psychosomatic disorders. The place of sleep and dreams revisited'. *Psychotherapy and Psychosomatics*, 1976, 27, 65–75.

Watts, G. O. *Dynamic Neuroscience*, New York: Harper, 1975.

Wilkinson, M. *Living with Migraine*, London: Heinemann, 1976.

If your local library hasn't got any of the above, ask the librarian to order them for you.

GENERAL NON-FICTION

0352303018	Godfrey Baseley **A COUNTRY COMPENDIUM**	£1.50
0352301392	Linda Blandford **OIL SHEIKHS**	95p
0352396121	Anthony Cave Brown **BODYGUARD OF LIES (Large Format)**	£2.50*
Δ 0352302925	**CLOSE ENCOUNTERS OF THE THIRD KIND**	95p*
035230345X	Rodney Dale and Joan Gray **EDWARDIAN INVENTIONS**	£2.95
0352301368	John Dean **BLIND AMBITION**	£1.50*
0352300124	Dr Fitzhugh Dodson **HOW TO PARENT**	75p*
0426190009	Trevor Donald **CONFESSIONS OF IDI AMIN**	95p†
0427004349	L. Grant **THE BASIC BABY BOOK**	95p
0352303247	H. R. Haldeman **THE ENDS OF POWER**	£1.25*
0352302674	Paul Hammond and Patrick Hughes **UPON THE PUN (illus)**	£1.25
0352303506	Clive Harold **THE UNINVITED**	95p
0426168623	Xaviera Hollander **THE HAPPY HOOKER**	80p*
0426163443	**LETTERS TO THE HAPPY HOOKER**	80p*
0426166787	**XAVIERA ON THE BEST PART OF A MAN**	80p*
0426134265	**XAVIERA!**	80p*
0352303891	Anne Fletcher **THE HAPPY HOOKER GOES TO WASHINGTON (F)**	90p*
0352305010	Francis Huxley **THE WAY OF THE SACRED**	£2.50*
Δ 0352304227	Paul Scanlon and Michael Gross **THE BOOK OF ALIEN**	£1.95*
0352301627	Sharon Lawrence **SO YOU WANT TO BE A ROCK & ROLL STAR**	95p*
0426087232	David Lewis **SEXPIONAGE**	70p
0426087151	**THE SECRET LIFE OF ADOLF HITLER**	75p

† For sale in Britain and Ireland only.
* Not for sale in Canada. ● Reissues.
Δ Film & T.V. tie-ins.

GENERAL NON-FICTION

0426086945	Linda Lovelace **THE INTIMATE DIARY OF** **LINDA LOVELACE**	60p
0426187458	Matthew Manning **IN THE MINDS OF MILLIONS**	95p*
0352302704	Peter Mayle **WILL I LIKE IT? (large format illus)**	£1.95*
0352304790	Judith Midgley-Carver and Amanda Duckett **CAREER CHOICES**	70p
035239692X	Henry Miller **THE WORLD OF SEX**	60p
0427004284	Jay Robert Nash **DARKEST HOURS (Large Format)**	£5.00
0352306165	Michael Nicholson **THE YORKSHIRE RIPPER**	95p
0426086007	Gerard I. Nievenberg & Henry H. Calero **HOW TO READ A PERSON LIKE A BOOK**	95p
0426175158	Sakuzawa Nyoiti **MACROBIOTICS**	50p*
0426186303	Sean O'Callahagn **THE TRIADS**	85p
0352302151	Molly Parkin **GOOD GOLLY MS MOLLY** (see also under General Fiction)	£1.25
0352301449	J. B. Priestley **MAN AND TIME**	£1.50*
0352395311	Neville Randall & Gary Keane **FOCUS ON FACT:** **THE WORLD OF INVENTION (illus)**	75p
035239532X	**THE STORY OF SPORT (illus)**	75p
035239529X	**THE PSYCHIC WORLD (illus)**	75p
0352395303	**THE STORY OF CHRISTMAS (illus)**	75p
0352395338	**UNSOLVED MYSTERIES (illus)**	75p
0352395346	**THE STORY OF FLIGHT (illus)**	75p
0426181638	Suze Randall **SUZE**	75p*
Δ 0352302410	Esther Rantzen **THAT'S LIFE (Large Format)**	£1.95
0352398639	Donald Rumbelow **THE COMPLETE JACK THE RIPPER**	£1.25

† For sale in Britain and Ireland only.
* Not for sale in Canada. ● Reissues.
Δ Film & T.V. tie-ins.

GENERAL FICTION

Δ	042697114X	Cyril Abraham **THE ONEDIN LINE: THE SHIPMASTER**	80p
Δ	0426132661	**THE ONEDIN LINE: THE IRON SHIPS**	80p
Δ	042616184X	**THE ONEDIN LINE: THE HIGH SEAS**	80p
Δ	0426172671	**THE ONEDIN LINE: THE TRADE WINDS**	80p
Δ	0352304006	**THE ONEDIN LINE: THE WHITE SHIPS**	95p
	0352302550	Spiro T. Agnew **THE CANFIELD DECISION**	£1.25*
	0352302690	Lynne Reid Banks **MY DARLING VILLAIN**	85p
	0352304251	T. G. Barclay **A SOWER WENT FORTH**	£1.95
Δ	0352302747	Michael J. Bird **THE APHRODITE INHERITANCE**	85p
	0352302712	Judy Blume **FOREVER**	75p*
Δ	0352305355	John Brason **SECRET ARMY: THE END OF THE LINE**	75p
	0352303441	Barbara Brett **BETWEEN TWO ETERNITIES**	75p*
	0352305916	André Brink **RUMOURS OF RAIN**	£1.95
	0352302003	Jeffrey Caine **HEATHCLIFF**	75p
	0352395168	**THE COLD ROOM**	85p
	0352304987	Ramsey Campbell **THE DOLL WHO ATE HIS MOTHER**	95p*
	0352305398	**THE FACE THAT MUST DIE**	95p
	0352300647	**DEMONS BY DAYLIGHT**	95p*

BARBARA CARTLAND'S ANCIENT WISDOM SERIES

	0427004209	Barbara Cartland **THE FORGOTTEN CITY**	70p*
	0427004217	L. Adams Beck **THE HOUSE OF FULFILMENT**	70p*
	0427004225	Marie Corelli **A ROMANCE OF TWO WORLDS**	70p*
	0427004233	Talbot Mundy **BLACK LIGHT**	70p*
	0427004241	L. Adams Beck **THE GARDEN OF VISION**	70p*

† For sale in Britain and Ireland only.
* Not for sale in Canada. ● Reissues.
Δ Film & T.V. tie-ins.

Wyndham Books are obtainable from many booksellers and newsagents. If you have any difficulty please send purchase price plus postage on the scale below to:

Wyndham Cash Sales
P.O. Box 11
Falmouth
Cornwall
OR
Star Book Service,
G.P.O. Box 29,
Douglas,
Isle of Man,
British Isles.

While every effort is made to keep prices low, it is sometimes necessary to increase prices at short notice. Wyndham Books reserve the right to show new retail prices on covers which may differ from those advertised in the text or elsewhere.

Postage and Packing Rate

UK: 30p for the first book, plus 15p per copy for each additional book ordered to a maximum charge of £1.29. **BFPO and Eire:** 30p for the first book, plus 15p per copy for the next 6 books and thereafter 6p per book. **Overseas:** 50p for the first book and 15p per copy for each additional book.

These charges are subject to Post Office charge fluctuations.